Medical Interpreting

NEW TRENDS IN TRANSLATION STUDIES

Volume 38

Series Editor:
Professor Jorge Díaz Cintas

Advisory Board:
Professor Susan Bassnett
Professor Lynne Bowker
Professor Frederic Chaume
Professor Aline Remael

PETER LANG
Oxford - Berlin - Bruxelles - Chennai - Lausanne - New York

Medical Interpreting

Training the Professionals

Almudena Nevado Llopis and
Ana Isabel Foulquié Rubio (eds)

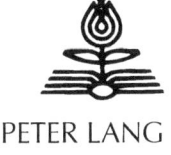

PETER LANG

Oxford - Berlin - Bruxelles - Chennai - Lausanne - New York

Bibliographic information published by the Deutsche Nationalbibliothek.
The German National Library lists this publication in the German National
Bibliography; detailed bibliographic data is available on the Internet at
http://dnb.d-nb.de.

A catalogue record for this book is available from the British

Library of Congress Cataloging-in-Publication Data

Names: Llopis, Almudena Nevado, 1976– editor. | Foulquié-Rubio,
   Ana-Isabel, editor.
Title: Medical interpreting : training the professionals / Almudena Nevado
   Llopis and Ana Isabel Foulquié Rubio, [editors].
Description: Oxford ; New York : Peter Lang, [2024] | Series: New trends in
   translation studies, 1664-249X ; volume no. 38 | Includes
   bibliographical references and index.
Identifiers: LCCN 2023047436 (print) | LCCN 2023047437 (ebook) |
   ISBN 9781800793217 (paperback) | ISBN 9781800793224 (ebook) |
   ISBN 9781800793231 (epub)
Subjects: LCSH: Medicine—Translating. | Health facilities—Translating
   services. | Medicine—Translating—Spain. |
   Medicine—Translating—Italy. | Medicine—Translating—Romania. | Health
   facilities—Translating services—Spain. | Health
   facilities—Translating services—Italy. | Health
   facilities—Translating services—Romania.
Classification: LCC R119.5 .M43 2024 (print) | LCC R119.5 (ebook) | DDC
   610.1/4—dc23/eng/20240102
LC record available at https://lccn.loc.gov/2023047436
LC ebook record available at https://lccn.loc.gov/2023047437

Co-funded by the Erasmus+ programme of the European Union.
Cover design by Peter Lang Group AG

ISSN 1664-249X
ISBN 978-1-80079-321-7 (print)
ISBN 978-1-80079-322-4 (ePDF)
ISBN 978-1-80079-323-1 (ePub)
DOI 10.3726/b18108

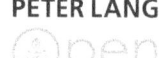 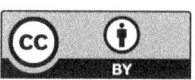

Open Access: This work is licensed under a Creative Commons Attribution CC-BY 4.0 license. To
view a copy of this license, visit https://creativecommons.org/licenses/by/4.0/

© 2024 Almudena Nevado Llopis and Ana Isabel Foulquié Rubio
Published by Peter Lang Ltd, Oxford, United Kingdom
info@peterlang.com – www.peterlang.com

Almudena Nevado Llopis and Ana Isabel Foulquié Rubio have asserted their right under the Copyright,
Designs and Patents Act, 1988, to be identified as Editors of this Work.

This publication has been peer reviewed.

Contents

List of Figures   vii

List of Tables   ix

RAQUEL LÁZARO GUTIÉRREZ
Foreword   xi

ALMUDENA NEVADO LLOPIS AND ANA ISABEL FOULQUIÉ RUBIO
Introducing the ReACTMe Project: Past, Present and Future   1

ANA ISABEL FOULQUIÉ RUBIO, NATACHA NIEMANTS AND ALINA ANDREICA
1   Medical Interpreting in Spain, Italy and Romania: Healthcare Providers' and Users' Viewpoints   9

ALMUDENA NEVADO LLOPIS, FRANCESCA GNANI AND ALINA PELEA
2   Medical Interpreter Training in Spain, Italy and Romania: State of Affairs and Expectations for the Future   57

ANA ISABEL FOULQUIÉ RUBIO, DONATELLA CIFOLA AND VERONICA MANOLE
3   Suggestions for the Professionalization of Medical Interpreting in Spain, Italy and Romania   103

ELEONORA BERNARDI AND LINDSEY BRUTON
4   Training Resources and Methodologies for Medical Interpreters   127

CHRISTOPHER GARWOOD
5 Key Elements to Be Considered When Designing a Course for Medical Interpreters — 153

ELENA TOMASSINI
6 A Model Joint Blended-Learning Module for Medical Interpreters — 165

BEVERLY COSTA
7 Reflective Practice Support for Interpreters: Why, What and How? — 185

CYNTHIA E. ROAT
8 Reweaving the Tapestry: How Healthcare Interpreters Will Save the World — 201

ANA ISABEL FOULQUIÉ RUBIO
Annex. Guidelines for Working with Medical Interpreters — 219

Notes on Contributors — 229

Index — 235

Figures

Figure 4.1.	ReACTMe learning platform: English resources for the development of cultural and intercultural competences	132
Figure 4.2.	ReACTMe platform: example of training resources 'index card'	133
Figure 4.3.	Case study 8. Misunderstanding about the gravity of the diagnosis	139
Figure 4.4.	Scripted roleplay from the ReACTMe First Intensive Programme for Higher Education Learners on Medical Interpreting	144
Figure 4.5.	Semi or unscripted roleplay from the First Intensive Programme for Higher Education Learners	145
Figure A.1.	English guidelines for working with medical interpreters	221
Figure A.2.	Spanish poster with QR code to access guidelines for working with medical interpreters	222
Figure A.3.	Spanish guidelines for working with medical interpreters	223
Figure A.4.	Italian poster with QR code to access guidelines for working with medical interpreters	224
Figure A.5.	Italian guidelines for working with medical interpreters	225
Figure A.6.	Romanian poster with QR code to access guidelines for working with medical interpreters	226
Figure A.7.	Romanian guidelines for working with medical interpreters	227

Tables

Table 1.1.	Questions for year 1 and year 3	11
Table 1.2.	Interviews carried out in each country classified by year and target population	14
Table 2.1.	Courses related to medical interpreting offered at Spanish universities	62
Table 2.2.	Languages studied within degree programmes in translation and interpreting in Spain	65
Table 2.3.	Country of origin of the fifteen largest foreign communities living in Spain	67
Table 2.4.	Foreign citizens living in Italy (aged 6 or above) according to their first language	74
Table 2.5.	Interpreting and translation-related degrees at UniBuc, UBB and UTCB	78
Table 6.1.	Programme of the Joint Blended Extracurricular Module	166
Table 6.2.	Competences to be developed by the students attending the module and their associated learning outcomes	174

RAQUEL LÁZARO GUTIÉRREZ

Foreword

The needs of our modern superdiverse societies have set the ground for the emergence and consolidation of new knowledge areas, research disciplines and professional figures (Vertovec 2007). Multiculturality and multilingualism are two of the main characteristics of contemporary societies, and communication is acknowledged as essential for healthy conviviality, inclusivity and sustainability in communities of all kinds, as reflected in the description of the UN Sustainable Development Goals (<https://sdgs.un.org/goals>). Equal and efficient public service provision for all implies dealing with barriers to access in an effective way, and interpreters, in the broadest sense of the word, have been considered key agents in this task (Lázaro Gutiérrez and Tejero González 2022).

It is true that interpreting studies have grown exponentially over the years, and this is a clear sign of consolidation for both a knowledge area and a research discipline that is intimately connected to the needs of superdiverse societies. Ever-increasing population movements and interactions, which are no longer exclusively physical but are also giving way to hybrid and virtual modalities, put communication in the spotlight. Multilingual institutional interactions in the domain of public service provision are increasingly the object of research in the field of translation and interpreting studies. In particular, research into medical interpreting has been addressed in several monographs published during the last two decades: Montalt i Resurrecció and Shuttleworth (2012), Varela Salinas and Meyer (2015) and Ji et al. (2019), combining interpreting and translation; or Pöchhacker and Shlesinger (2005), Andres and Pöllabauer (2009), Lázaro Gutiérrez (2012), Nicodemus and Metzger (2014) and Souza and Fragkou (2020), dealing exclusively with interpreting.

One of the most salient topics in publications on public service interpreting in general, and medical interpreting in particular, is that of professionalization. Lázaro Gutiérrez and Gauthier Blasi (2020) reflect upon the professionalization of medical interpreters and, importantly, their role as change agents in modern societies. The authors' work is based on the sociological work of Spencer (1992), who states that all structures in society arise from the specialization of a relatively homogeneous group. This specialization generates knowledge, which is transformed into symbolic capital and thus strengthens the group by giving it a certain symbolic power. Besides, from a business and financial point of view, generators and indicators of power have changed from the possession of land and the production of material goods to the possession of specialization and the production of knowledge. This change is due, in part, to the democratization of access to university education for the former working class of the industrial era. As the acquisition of power in modern societies is based on specialized knowledge, professions turn into new power elites, and each group of professionals struggles to activate and impose its symbolic capital in order to ensure its recognition and permanence (Bourdieu 1986). In the case of public service interpreting in general and medical interpreting in particular, the sociology of professions also informs us that an orientation towards the well-being of society is one of the minimal characteristics and requirements of professions, as they intend to contribute to social improvement and progress (Rodríguez Ávila 2008: 17). This volume constitutes one of the outcomes of the ReACTMe project and presents a range of interesting contributions on the social role of medical interpreters, the status of their professionalization and their training in several European countries.

In the literature related to professionalization, references to training are very prominent and education is considered one of the main elements of professionalization (Harries-Jenkins 1979). Specialized and theoretical knowledge is paramount to delimit professional practical skills (Wilensky 1964; Evetts 2003; Panaia 2007; Nolin 2008). This knowledge is transmitted and acquired through extensive training at university level or in specialized training schools (Goode 1957; Wilensky 1964; Lázaro Gutiérrez and Álvaro Aranda 2020), which also provide graduates with certification and professional status (Paradeise 1984; Burrage et al. 1990). In highly professionalized activities, such certification implies a sine qua non condition to access employment (Paradeise 1984).

Given the current professional status of medical interpreting, still fighting for full professionalization, it is not surprising that much of the scientific research in medical interpreting has revolved around interpreters' competences and training needs. This has been addressed from a pedagogical point of view in the shape of manuals for the training or self-training of interpreters, such as Abraham et al. (2004), Swabey and Malcolm (2012), Valero Garcés (2014), Bancroft et al. (2016) and Angelelli (2019), or the series by Crezee et al. (2013, 2015, 2016), oriented towards the development of interpreters' thematic competence, that is, knowledge about healthcare. The literature also provides us with descriptions of innovative teaching and learning practices, such as the work of Niemants and Stokoe (2017), who apply the CARM (Conversation Analytic Roleplay Method) developed by Stokoe (2014) to train Italian–French medical interpreters, or that of Dal Fovo (2018), who contrasts the usefulness in the classroom of the observation and discussion of examples from two different corpora, one containing authentic doctor-patient interactions and another consisting of simulations. Another pedagogical experiment based on situated learning is that carried out by Sanz Moreno (2017), who invited healthcare professionals into the interpreting classroom to practice with roleplays and discuss codes of ethics with interpreting students. Hlavac and Harrison (2021) took a similar approach using the interprofessional education (IPE) strategy, widely used in healthcare training, which consists of structured and mainly situation-based training that involves two or more groups of professionals. Other examples of interprofessional training have been carried out in Belgium, by Krystallidou et al. (2018), and Italy, by Gattiglia and Morelli (2022).

We can also see the impact of the technological turn on medical interpreting training, particularly in the prevalence of studies incorporating the use of corpus tools. For instance, Sánchez Ramos (2017) uses corpus analysis to train interpreters and develop their documentation skills, and Major and McKee (2020) carry out a terminological study with a corpus of deaf New Zealand Sign Language users' accounts of women's health-related experiences to identify vocabulary and language forms to be included in interpreter training. Also related to new technologies are different training proposals that focus on remote interpreting modalities (over the phone and through video link), such as Albl-Mikasa and Eingrieber (2018) with a proposal to train interpreters who work using video link, or the 'SHIFT in Orality' project (Amato et al. 2018), and a revolutionary proposal by Eser et al. (2020), who describe a learning experience based on the use of three-dimensional virtual reality glasses to train medical interpreters in immersive simulated environments.

In fact, the main asset of the ReACTMe project is its success in the development of training materials for interpreter trainers and the design of innovative, comprehensive and transferable training modules for medical interpreters. The project's focus on research into the current situation in terms of the needs, services and training is paramount to contributing to the professionalization of medical interpreting. Ultimately, the results and outcomes that have emerged, and continue to emerge, from ReACTMe will go a long way towards covering urgent necessities in the field and with the clear motivation to satisfy those of the scientific and the professional communities around medical interpreting.

Bibliography

Abraham, Diana, Nelson Cabral, and Anita Tancredi (eds). 2004. *A Handbook for Trainers: Language Interpreting in the Healthcare Sector*. Toronto: Healthcare Interpretation Network.

Albl-Mikasa, Michaela, and Monika Eingrieber. 2018. 'Training video interpreters for refugee languages in the German-speaking DACH countries', *FITISPos International Journal* 5, 33–44.

Amato, Amalia, Nicoletta Spinolo, and María Jesús González Rodríguez (eds). 2018. *Handbook of Remote Interpreting – SHIFT in Orality*. Bologna: University of Bologna.

Andres, Dörte, and Sonja Pöllabauer (eds). 2009. *Spürst Du, wie der Bauch raufrunter? Fachdolmetschen im Gesundheitsbereich: Is Everything All Topsy Turvy in Your Tummy? Healthcare Interpreting*. Munich: Meidenbauer.

Angelelli, Claudia V. 2019. *Healthcare Interpreting Explained*. London: Routledge.
Bancroft, Marjory A., Sofia Garcia Beyaert, Katharine Allen, Giovanna Carriero-Contreras, and Denis Socarras-Estrada. 2016. *The Medical Interpreter: A Foundation Textbook for Medical Interpreting*. Columbia: Culture & Language Press.
Bourdieu, Pierre. 1986. 'The forms of capital', in John G. Richardson (ed.), *Handbook of Theory and Research for the Sociology of Education*. Westport, CT: Greenwood, 241–258.
Burrage, Michael, Konrad Jarausch, and Hannes Seigrist. 1990. 'An actor-based framework for the study of the professions', in Michael Burrage and Rolf Torstendahl (eds), *Professions in Theory and History: Rethinking the Study of the Professions*. London.: Sage, 203–225.
Crezee, Ineke. 2013. *Introduction to Healthcare for Interpreters and Translators*. Amsterdam: John Benjamins.
Crezee, Ineke, and Eva N. S. Ng. 2016. *Introduction to Healthcare for Chinese-Speaking Interpreters and Translators*. Amsterdam: John Benjamins.
Crezee, Ineke, Holly Mikkelson, and Laura Monzon-Storey. 2015. *Introduction to Healthcare for Spanish-Speaking Interpreters and Translators*. Amsterdam: John Benjamins.
Crezee, Ineke, Nawar Gailani, and Anna N. Gailani. 2016. *Introduction to Healthcare for Arabic-speaking Interpreters and Translators*. Amsterdam: John Benjamins.
Dal Fovo, Eugenia. 2018. 'The use of dialogue interpreting corpora in healthcare interpreter training: Taking stock', *The Interpreters' Newsletter* 23, 83–113.
Eser, Oktay, Miranda Lai, and Fatih Saltan. 2020. 'The affordances and challenges of wearable technologies for training public service interpreters', *Interpreting* 22(2), 288–308.
Evetts, Julia. 2003. 'The sociological analysis of professionalism: Occupational change in the modern world', *International Sociology* 18(2), 395–415.
Gattiglia, Nora, and Mara Morelli. 2022. *Comunicazione multilinguistica in ambito sanitario: Curare e riflettere tra lingue, culture e mediazioni*. Genoa: Genova University Press.
Goode, William J. 1957. 'Community within a community: The professions', *American Sociological Review* 22(2), 194–200.
Harries-Jenkins, Gwyn. 1979. *The Army in Victorian Society*. London: Routledge.
Hlavac, Jim, and Claire Harrison. 2021. 'Interpreter-mediated doctor-patient interactions: Interprofessional education in the training of future interpreters and doctors', *Perspectives* 29(4), 572–590.
Ji, Meng, Mustapha Taibi, and Ineke Crezee (eds). 2019. *Multicultural Health Translation, Interpreting and Communication*. London: Routledge.

Krystallidou, Demi, Céline Van De Walle, Myriam Deveugele, Evangelia Dougali, Fien Mertens, Amélie Truwant, Ellen Van Praet, and Peter Pype. 2018. 'Training "doctor-minded" interpreters and "interpreter-minded" doctors: The benefits of collaborative practice in interpreter training', *Interpreting* 20(1), 132–150.

Lázaro Gutiérrez, Raquel. 2012. *La interpretación en el ámbito sanitario: estudio de la asimetría en consultas médicas*. Saarbrücken: Editorial Académica Española, LAP LAMBERT Academic Publishing.

Lázaro Gutiérrez, Raquel, and Cristina Álvaro Aranda. 2020. 'Public service interpreting and translation in Spain', in Marketa Štefková, Koen Kerremans, and Benjamin Bossaert (eds), *Training Public Service Interpreters and Translators: A European Perspective*. Bratislava: Univerzita Komenského v Bratislave.

Lázaro Gutiérrez, Raquel, and Laura Gauthier Blasi. 2020. 'Vers la professionnalisation de l'interprétation en milieu de soins de santé: Quel degré d'(in)visibilité pour l'interprète?' *The Interpreters' Newsletter* 25, 81–94.

Lázaro Gutiérrez, Raquel, and Jesús Manuel Tejero González. 2022. 'Challenging ideologies and fostering intercultural competence: The discourses of healthcare staff about linguistic and cultural barriers, interpreters, and mediators', in Simo Määttä and Marika K. Hall (eds), *Mapping Ideology in Discourse Studies*. Berlin: De Gruyter Mouton, 223–246.

Major, George, and Rachel McKee. 2000. 'Deaf women's health vocabulary: Challenges for interpreters working in a language of limited diffusion', *International Journal of Interpreter Education (IJIE)* 12(2), 1–18.

Montalt i Resurrecció, Vicent, and Mark Shuttleworth (eds). 2012. 'Research in translation and knowledge mediation in medical and healthcare settings', *Linguistica Antverpiensia, New Series* 11.

Nicodemus, Brenda, and Melanie Metzger (eds). 2014. *Investigations in Healthcare Interpreting*. Washington, DC: Gallaudet University.

Niemants, Natascha, and Elizabeth Stokoe. 2017. 'Using the conversation analytic role-play method in healthcare interpreter education', in Letizia Cirillo and Natacha Niemants (eds), *Teaching Dialogue Interpreting: Research-Based Proposals for Higher Education*. Amsterdam: John Benjamins, 294–321.

Nolin, Jan. 2008. *In Search of a New Theory of Professions*. Boras: University of Boras.

Panaia, Marta. 2007. *Una revisión de la sociología de las profesiones desde la teoría crítica del trabajo en la Argentina*. Santiago de Chile: CEPAL.

Paradeise, Catherine. 1984. 'La marine marchande: un marché du travail fermé?', *Revue française de sociologie* XXV(3), 352–375.

Pöchhacker, Franz, and Miriam Shlesinger (eds). 2005. 'Healthcare interpreting: Discourse and interaction', *Interpreting* 7(2).

Rodríguez Avila, Nuria. 2008. *Manual de sociología de las profesiones*. Barcelona: University of Barcelona.
Sánchez Ramos, María del Mar. 2017. 'Interpretación sanitaria y herramientas informáticas de traducción: los sistemas de gestión de corpus', *Panace@* 18(46), 133–141.
Sanz-Moreno, Raquel. 2017. 'Dilemas éticos en interpretación sanitaria: El médico entra en el aula', *Panace@* 18(46), 114–122.
Souza, Isabel, and Effrossyni Fragkou (eds). 2022. *Handbook of Research on Medical Interpreting*. Hershey: IGI Global.
Spencer, Herbert. 1992. 'El origen de las profesiones', *Reis: Revista española de investigaciones sociológicas* 59, 317–328.
Stokoe, Elizabeth. 2014. 'The conversation analytic role-play method (CARM): A method for training communication skills as an alternative to simulated role-play', *Research on Language and Social Interaction* 47, 255–265.
Swabey, Laurie, and Karen Malcolm (eds). 2012. *In Our Hands: Educating Healthcare Interpreters*. Washington, DC: Gallaudet University.
Valero-Garcés, Carmen. 2014. *Health, Communication and Multicultural Communities: Topics on Intercultural Communication for Healthcare Professionals*. Newcastle upon Tyne: Cambridge Scholars Publishing.
Varela Salinas, María-José, and Bernd Meyer (eds). 2015. *Translating and Interpreting Healthcare Discourses / Traducir e interpretar en el ámbito sanitario*. Berlin: Frank & Timme.
Vertovec, Steven. 2007. 'Super-diversity and its implications', *Ethnic and Racial Studies* 30(6), 1024–1054.
Wilensky, Harold, L. 1964. 'The professionalization of everyone?', *American Journal of Sociology* 707(2), 137–158.

ALMUDENA NEVADO LLOPIS AND ANA ISABEL FOULQUIÉ RUBIO

Introducing the ReACTMe Project: Past, Present and Future

The ReACTMe project, a three-year Erasmus+ project,[1] set out on its journey in September 2019 with the deep and heartfelt enthusiasm of all the team members. The project consortium was made up of six universities from three countries: Universidad San Jorge and Universidad de Murcia from Spain, Università di Bologna and Università degli Studi Internazionali di Roma from Italy, and Universitatea Babeș-Bolyai and Universitatea de Medicină și Farmacie Iuliu Hațieganu from Romania.

ReACTMe's main objective was to improve medical interpreter training in the participating countries and consequently to contribute to ensuring effective communication between healthcare providers and foreign-language-speaking patients. We started from the premise that, as stated in previous studies (Wynia and Osborn 2010; Vermeir et al. 2015; Merlino 2017; Ratna 2019), access to and quality of healthcare is only possible if the key players in the healthcare setting are able to communicate successfully.

Despite evidence of the negative effects that linguistic and cultural barriers can have on the healthcare provided to allophone patients (migrants, refugees, tourists, visitors and international students), in many European countries, including Spain, Italy and Romania, these barriers were – and unfortunately still are – frequently overcome using family members or friends and other non-professional (ad hoc) interpreters. Although in some cases patients may feel more at ease (Zendelel et al. 2018), such interpreters may perform poorly, which can have a clinically significant impact on patient care (Flores et al. 2003; Meyer et al. 2010; Kilian et al. 2014). In our

---

1   Project number 2019-1-ES01-KA203-064439.

opinion, the use of ad hoc medical interpreters is to a large extent related to a lack of medical interpreting training programmes and certification and accreditation processes of medical interpreters. In this respect, European higher education institutions have a great responsibility to provide innovative and specialized training for medical interpreters, to help them acquire and develop the necessary skills, knowledge and attitudes to overcome the linguistic and cultural barriers that allophone patients encounter when accessing and using healthcare services. In summary, with this project we expected the participating higher education institutions to contribute to the professionalization of medical interpreting, and in this way encourage the promotion of equality and social inclusion in healthcare.

The ReACTMe project has addressed linguistic and cultural diversity and tried to promote equality, non-discrimination and social inclusion through training at higher education level. In particular, we aimed to foster the development of medical interpreting as a profession requiring specialized training, not only amongst participant students and trainers but also amongst key stakeholders and policy/decision makers at the local, regional and national levels in all the participating countries. Additionally, our intention was to tackle discrimination in healthcare and promote the use of professional medical interpreters through the undertaking of research in this area, and the subsequent creation of a learning platform, the design of a curriculum for a joint blended-learning module on medical interpreting, and the development of two sets of guidelines: one for teaching and learning medical interpreting on the one hand, and one for working with medical interpreters on the other.

With these aims in mind, research and action methodology, understood as 'a form of collective self-reflective enquiry undertaken by participants in social situations in order to improve the rationality and justice of their own social or educational practices, as well as their understanding of these practices and the situations in which these practices are carried out' (Kemmis and McTaggart 1988: 1), seemed to be the most appropriate. Therefore, we followed this methodology over the three years of the project to produce changes progressively and cyclically, firstly in universities and then in societies and healthcare services and societies. In this way, the ReACTMe researchers have been part of societal change and helped raise awareness about the relevance of training and professionalization of medical interpreters.

In short, through training in universities, we wanted to take the necessary steps to provide the resources for well-trained medical interpreters working with Spanish, Italian and Romanian as well as other European languages in each of the three participating countries. In line with the above, actions, methodology and outputs were designed to:

- allow the project team to draw a clear and realistic picture of the current situation of medical interpreting in Spain, Italy and Romania;
- pilot the delivery of existing and newly developed content and teaching and learning materials on medical interpreting;
- train both higher education trainers and students on medical interpreting.

The main results obtained in the ReACTMe project are described in this volume,[2] which is composed of eight chapters, six of which are devoted to results of the research carried out by the team members (Chapters 1–6). The two last chapters are written by researchers with long experience in this field who participated either in the final international conference of the project or in the ReACTMe newsletter quarterly published from April 2020 to July 2022. Additionally, there is one Annex in which one of the intellectual outputs developed during the project is presented.

Chapters 1–6 deal directly with the results of the ReACTMe project. Chapter 1, 'Medical Interpreting in Spain, Italy and Romania: Healthcare Providers' and Users' Viewpoints' by Ana Isabel Foulquié Rubio, Natacha Niemants and Alina Andreica, deals with the results of the research conducted in years 1 and 3 of the ReACTMe project. During year 1 (2019–2020), policy and decision makers were interviewed to learn about their perspective on the current situation of medical interpreting and the existing legislation, if any, related to the support of allophone patients. In this first

---

2   The project, as well as this volume, have been co-funded by the Erasmus+ programme of the European Union.

year, the perspectives of members of NGOs and professional associations were also collected. During year 3 (2021–2022), frontline healthcare professionals and allophone patients were interviewed to learn about their experiences and opinions regarding their communication with each other. In short, Chapter 1 provides a clear overview of the situation of medical interpreting in the three participating countries from the point of view of those directly involved. It also offers evidence of the need to work with different key players in these settings to make them aware of the importance of professional interpreting when providing quality healthcare services.

Chapter 2, 'Medical Interpreter Training in Spain, Italy and Romania: State of Affairs and Expectations for the Future' by Almudena Nevado Llopis, Francesca Gnani and Alina Pelea, is dedicated to a comparison of the situation of medical interpreter training in the three countries. To achieve an overview of the situation, during year 2 of the research (2020–2021), researchers conducted a document analysis and a literature review and organized different focus groups with professional (medical) interpreters, higher education representatives, and translation and interpreting trainers. This chapter also analyses the medical interpreter training provided in Spanish, Italian and Romanian universities, illustrating the need for specialized training, and explores the competences required for interpreting in healthcare settings, as well as the most adequate methods and resources to acquire and develop those competences.

In Chapter 3, 'Suggestions for the Professionalization of Medical Interpreting in Spain, Italy and Romania', Ana Isabel Foulquié Rubio, Donatella Cifola and Veronica Manole deal with the issue of professionalization and its importance for the recognition of and institutional support for medical interpreting. The chapter is based on both the information gathered during the three years of project and the analysis of the current situation of medical interpreting in the three participating countries extracted from the literature review.

Eleonora Bernardi and Lindsey Bruton are authors of Chapter 4, 'Training Resources and Methodologies for Medical Interpreters', which, as can be inferred by its title, examines the resources and methodologies that can best be applied to the training of medical interpreters. They present and take as a reference the Learning Platform created as one of the outputs of the ReACTMe project. As will be explained in the chapter, the platform provides trainers and students of medical interpreting, as well as professional interpreters, with different resources such as roleplays, terminology activities, case studies, a compilation of online resources on different languages organized according to key competences and a multilingual glossary of specialized terminology structured by health specializations.

Chapter 5, 'Key Elements to Be Considered when Designing a Course for Medical Interpreters', authored by Christopher Garwood, presents the Guidelines and Training Resources for Teaching/Learning Medical Interpreting that can be found in the ReACTMe Learning Platform, which contain useful information about the considerations to be made before designing a course on medical interpreting, the most adequate course structure and organization, and some suggested teaching and learning materials to be used in such a course.

The last chapter authored by the ReACTMe researchers is Chapter 6, 'A Model Joint Blended Learning Module for Medical Interpreters', written by Elena Tomassini, focuses on the Joint Blended Extracurricular Module on Medical Interpreting developed within the project. It includes its programme, competences and learning outcomes, as well as contents and examples of materials for a future programme for training medical interpreters that will be implemented at the partner universities and could be adapted to suit the needs and characteristics of other educational institutions.

Chapter 7, 'Reflective Practice Support for Interpreters – Why, What and How?' authored by Beverly Costa, deals with the emotional support that medical interpreters need. The author proposes reflective practice support and discusses the way such assistance is delivered. Costa also proposes the need to train interpreters to act as facilitators who may deliver this support and briefly presents the programme developed by the Pásalo Project.

In Chapter 8, 'Reweaving the Tapestry: How Healthcare Interpreters Will Save the World', Cynthia E. Roat offers an overview of the development of the medical interpreting profession in the United States. Roat comments on the different phases through which a profession needs to go to achieve full professionalization, and explains the different strategies that helped the development of the profession in the United States, such as convincing hospitals and clinics about the importance of using professional interpreters, improving research in the field, creating and applying legislation, organizing accreditation processes for professional interpreting, and using the press to inform the public about the situations that result from the use of non-professional interpreters.

Finally, the Annex presents the multilingual Guidelines for Working with Interpreters, which were developed after analysing information gathered during workshops for healthcare students and professionals organized by the team members. The Guidelines consist of a decalogue, in a very simple form, laying out the most important aspects that healthcare professionals should consider when working with interpreters in order to ensure successful communication.

Back in September 2019, we could not have imagined how far we would come, how rich our outputs would be, how many trainers and students would participate in our training activities, how many professionals would benefit from our workshops and guidelines, or how many actors in the field we would meet and interview. In the end, they were much more than expected. To cut a long story short, we believe that, as a result of this project, which has been an extremely enriching experience for all of its partners, we will have contributed to raising awareness about the importance of effective communication in healthcare settings and the positive consequences of using professional medical interpreters. In the future, we hope to continue working towards giving the best possible training to future and current interpreters working in healthcare settings and, in this way, contribute to the professionalization of medical interpreting.

Bibliography

Flores, Glenn, Michael Barton Laws, Sandra J. Mayo, Barry Zuckerman, Milagros Abreu, Leonardo Medina, and Eric Hardt. 2003. 'Errors in medical interpretation and their potential clinical consequences in pediatric encounters', *Pediatrics* 111(1), 6–14. <https://doi.org/10.1542/peds.111.1.6>.

Kemmis, Stephen, and Robin McTaggart. 1988. *The Action Research Planner* (3rd ed.). Geelong: Deakin University Press.

Kilian, Sanja, Leslie Swartz, Tessa Dowling, Mawande Dlali, and Bonginkosi Chiliza. 2014. 'The potential consequences of informal interpreting practices for assessment of patients in a South African psychiatric hospital', *Social Science and Medicine* 106, 159–167. <https://doi.org/10.1016/j.socscimed.2014.01.019>.

Merlino, James. 2017. 'Communication: A critical healthcare competency', *Patient Safety & Quality Healthcare*, 6 November. <www.psqh.com/analysis/communication-critical-healthcare-competency>.

Meyer, Bernd, Birte Pawlack, and Ortrun Kliche. 2010. 'Family interpreters in hospitals: Good reasons for bad practice?', *mediAzioni*, 10.

Ratna, Haran. 2019. 'The importance of effective communication in healthcare practice', *Harvard Public Health Review* 23, 1–6. <www.jstor.org/stable/48546767>.

Vermeir, Peter, Dominique Vandijck, Sophie Degroote, Renaat Peleman, Rik Verhaeghe, Eric Mortier, Giorgio Hallaert, Sabine Van Daele, William Buylaert, and Dirk Vogelaer. 2015. 'Communication in healthcare: A narrative review of the literature and practical recommendations', *The International Journal of Clinical Practice* 69(11), 1257–1267. <https://doi.org/10.1111/ijcp.12686>.

Wynia, Matthew K., and Chandra Y. Osborn. 2010. 'Health literacy and communication quality in health care organizations', *Journal of Health Communication* 15(2), 102–115. <https://doi.org/10.1080/10810730.2010.499981>.

Zendelel, Rena, Barbara C Schouten, Julia C M van Weert, and Bas van den Putte. 2018. 'Informal interpreting in general practice: Are interpreters' roles related to perceived control, trust, and satisfaction?', *Patient Education and Counseling* 101(6), 1058–1065. <https://doi.org/10.1016/j.pec.2018.01.012>.

ANA ISABEL FOULQUIÉ RUBIO, NATACHA NIEMANTS AND
ALINA ANDREICA

1 Medical Interpreting in Spain, Italy and Romania: Healthcare Providers' and Users' Viewpoints

1. Introduction

Medical interpreting mainly occurs in triadic exchanges in which patients and health professionals exchange information with the help of an interpreter. The role of the interpreter, however, is not always clear and can be shaped by the expectations of the other interlocutors in this exchange (Hsieh 2006; Sleptsova et al. 2015). For this reason, when trying to understand the phenomenon of medical interpreting, it is important to gather the opinions not only of interpreters but also of the professionals and patients who use interpreting services.

In this chapter, only the opinions and views of the primary participants in the exchange are analysed, leaving the third actor, the interpreter, for a separate chapter (see Chapter 2 in this volume) where the views of interpreters working in medical settings are analysed and presented.

According to Leanza (2005: 167), 'interpreting is more beneficial to the healthcare providers than to the patient'. For this reason, in this chapter we concentrate mainly on the opinions of healthcare providers, while also looking briefly at the experiences of healthcare users who, at the time of accessing the service, did not speak the official language of the country. The data collected in this study informs us about the expectations of the interpreter held by both parties, and about their experiences when no professional interpreting was provided.

2. Methodology

As explained in the introductory chapter of this volume, the ReACTMe project lasted three years (2019–2022) and addressed a variety of topics related to medical interpreting based on data collected from three participating countries: Italy, Romania and Spain. The information presented in this chapter corresponds to the research carried out during years 1 (2019–2020) and 3 (2021–2022) of the project. Different data-collection methods were used, and different target populations were addressed depending on the information being collected and the aim of each year.

The aim of year 1 was to assess the situation of medical interpreting provision and legislation, which was achieved by analysing the existing legislation in each country combining different methods such as a literature review and document analysis as well as information provided in personal interviews with the different stakeholders. During year 1, data was collected from policy decision makers, heads of department in hospitals and hospital managers on the one hand, as well as medical and patients' associations and NGOs working with migrant populations on the other.

The aim of year 3 was to evaluate the quality of medical interpreting services provided in the different countries according to the stakeholders. This was done by conducting interviews with people on the frontline of healthcare: healthcare providers communicating with allophone patients (HCPs) and allophone patients using healthcare services (HCUs).

The interviewees were selected using the above-mentioned target criteria in the three participating countries, and the data-collection method used was in-depth, semi-structured interviews. To ensure comparability of the collected data, the project team agreed on the questions and the interviews were first prepared in English, the working language throughout the project. The questions were then translated into the languages spoken by the interviewees in each country (i.e. Italian, Romanian and Spanish). The interview questions were presented to the ethics committee for each university (according to the requirements of each institution) and approval was granted. Interviewees were provided with a consent form to sign and an information sheet explaining the project.

Table 1.1. Questions for year 1 and year 3

Year 1	
Policy decision makers	Associations and NGOs
1. Is there any legislation ruling medical interpreting/mediation in Spain/Italy/Romania (or the specific region/city/hospital)? If so, please indicate the relevant pieces of legislation. 2. From the information you have, how are linguistic and cultural barriers between Spanish/Italian/Romanian healthcare providers and foreign-language-speaking patients overcome? 3. What would you expect from a medical interpreter/mediator? What are her/his role and her/his duties? 4. In your opinion, what are the main differences between non-professional (family members, friends, other patients, healthcare professionals) and professional medical interpreters/mediators? 5. (Only to hospital directors or heads of medical departments) As far as you know, have there been any problems at your workplace when using a non-professional/a professional medical interpreter/mediator? Could you describe that specific situation (who was involved, what the problem was, what consequences were derived, etc.)? (Closing: Would you like to add anything regarding this topic?)	1. (Only to medical/patient associations and NGOs representatives) Do healthcare professionals have difficulties when communicating with foreign-language-speaking patients? 2. (Only to medical/patient associations and NGOs representatives) How are these difficulties overcome? 3. Is there any legislation or regulation ruling medical interpreting in Spain/Italy/Romania (or the specific region/city/hospital)? If so, please indicate the relevant pieces of legislation. 4. (Only to interpreters' associations representatives) Is there any medical interpreters'/mediators' association in Spain/Italy/Romania? 5. (Only to interpreters' associations representatives) In case there aren't, do you think there should be at least one? Why? 6. (Only to interpreters' associations representatives) Is there any official code of ethics for medical interpreters/mediators in Spain/Italy/Romania? 7. What competences (knowledge, skills, attitudes) do you think a medical interpreter should have?

(continued)

Table 1.1.   Continued

Year 1	
Policy decision makers	Associations and NGOs
	8. What would you expect from a medical interpreter? What are her/his role and her/his duties? 9. In your opinion, what are the main differences between non-professional interpreters (family members, friends, other patients, healthcare professionals) and professional medical interpreters/mediators? (Closing: Would you like to add anything regarding this topic?)
Year 3	
Healthcare providers (doctors, nurses, helpdesk assistants, etc.)	Healthcare users
1. Do foreign-language-speaking patients use healthcare services at your workplace? 2. Do healthcare professionals at your workplace have difficulties when communicating with these patients? How are these difficulties overcome? 3. If there are professional interpreting services at your workplace, do the language combinations available answer the linguistic and cultural needs? 4. Are Spanish/Italian/Romanian healthcare providers and students informed about the interpreting services available (in case there are professional interpreting services)?	1. How are linguistic and cultural barriers between Spanish/Italian/Romanian healthcare providers and foreign-language-speaking patients overcome? 2. Do the language combinations available answer the linguistic and cultural needs in Spanish/Italian/Romanian healthcare services? 3. Are you, as a foreign-language-speaking patient, satisfied with the communication outcomes when using Spanish/Italian/Romanian healthcare services? 4. Have you had any problem when using an ad hoc medical interpreter (family members, friends, 'bilingual' medical staff, etc.)? Could you describe that specific situation (who was involved, what the problem was, what consequences were derived, etc.)?

Table 1.1. Continued

Year 1	
Policy decision makers	Associations and NGOs
5. Do you think that foreign-language-speaking patients are satisfied with the communication outcomes when they use Spanish/Italian/Romanian healthcare services? 6. As far as you know, have there been any problem at your workplace when using ad hoc medical interpreters (family members, friends, 'bilingual' medical staff, etc.)? Could you describe that specific situation (who was involved, what the problem was, what consequences were derived, etc.)? 7. Have you had any experiences with professional interpreters in healthcare settings? Could you briefly describe them stressing both the advantages and disadvantages of this collaboration? 8. Do you have suggestions for improving the quality of these services (from the point of view of logistics, skills, ethics, etc.)? (Closing: Would you like to add anything regarding this topic?)	5. Have you had any experiences with professional interpreters in healthcare settings? Could you briefly describe them stressing both the advantages and disadvantages of this collaboration? 6. Do you have suggestions for improving your communication as a foreign-language-speaking patient with the Spanish/Italian/Romanian healthcare professionals? (Closing: Would you like to add anything regarding this topic?)

Source: ReACTMe researchers

The interviews were carried out by the project team members in each country. Due to the COVID-19 pandemic, most of the interviews were carried out online using the available platforms. While this was an advantage in the sense that it allowed some interviewees to attend the interviews from greater distances, it may have caused people to feel less comfortable than they would have felt in face-to-face interviews. Despite this disadvantage, we were able to collect the necessary data.

Table 1.2. Interviews carried out in each country classified by year and target population

Country	Year 1		Year 3	
	Decision makers	Interpreters' associations & NGOs	Healthcare professionals	Patients
Spain	14	7	26	13
Italy	6	2	5	5
Romania	7	5	4	7

As for the number of participants, the aim at the initial stage of the ReACTMe project was to conduct at least three interviews per partner for year 1, and interviews with two healthcare professionals and two patients per partner for year 3. Even though the same number of interviews was not carried out in all participating countries, all three countries managed to conduct more interviews than the number required to fulfil the project aims, as shown in the table below:

The interviews reveal interesting results that allow us to achieve the goal of presenting a comparative analysis of the situation in the three countries (see Section 4).

All interviews were either audio or video recorded to allow the data to be analysed. The recordings were then transcribed and anonymized, and qualitative analysis was carried out. Nevertheless, it is important to consider that although the interviews were semi-structured, interviewers sometimes changed the order of the questions and interviewees were able to add additional information they considered important to the topic.

Each university analysed its own data, after which the analysed data were shared with the rest of the team of the project to compare the results, grouping the information by topic. Some of the results from year 1 have already been published in different publications (Tomassini et al. 2022; Garwood et al. 2023). This chapter, however, also includes the results from year 3 of the project and offers a comparative analysis of the results, depicting the situation not for each country in isolation but in comparison with the other countries participating in the project.

The data were analysed and compared according to the relevant stage of the project but also according to the different target groups. The information presented in Section 4 of this chapter is, therefore, divided according to the target groups.

3. The Spanish, Italian and Romanian healthcare systems

Health is a fundamental human right enshrined in international treaties and European conventions, and every member state that has ratified these conventions shall guarantee its enjoyment through national legislation and organizational choices. In all three participating countries – Spain, Italy and Romania – the right to access to healthcare services is guaranteed by their respective constitutions. To give specific information for each country, the right to access to healthcare services is guaranteed by the Spanish Constitution as well as by Law 16/2003 of 28 May. This law was modified by the Royal Decree-Law 7/2018 on Universal Access to the *Sistema Nacional de Salud* (National Health System 2018), which is granted to every Spanish citizen and those residing in Spain, including foreign regular/authorized and irregular/unauthorized populations. The Spanish healthcare system is also based on the Law on General Health, passed on 25 April 1986 (Law 14/1986 on General Health). In Italy, Article 32 of the Italian Constitution of 1948 states that health is a fundamental human right and ensures free access to healthcare to those who could otherwise not afford it, stressing the importance of respect for every individual in all circumstances. Articles 7 and 9 of the Charter of Values of Citizenship and Integration, adopted in 2007, complemented Article 32 of the Italian Constitution, underlining that this fundamental right to access to healthcare also applies to immigrants, who equally deserve medical treatment that fully respects their wishes, dignity and sensitivity (Gerolimich 2015). As is the case of Italy and Spain, the Constitution of Romania also mentions the right to healthcare. Article 34 guarantees the right to access to the Romanian healthcare services and Article 148 includes the obligation to respect the provisions and requirements of EU treaties in the domain of healthcare. Article 20 of the Constitution of Romania also includes the duty to respect human rights as part of the country's obligation to comply with the Universal Declaration of Human Rights, as well as with the international treaties and agreements to which the country is signatory (Constitution of Romania, Art. 20, 34, 148).

According to Ozolins (2000) and Giarelli (2008), the fact that healthcare is protected by a Constitution is not insignificant, because this influences the responses given by public and private institutions to the need of communication with allophone patients.

Unfortunately, however, 'the letter of the law cannot, by itself, guarantee the enjoyment of human rights in practice' (Vecchiato 2015: 11), especially when foreign patients do not speak the language of the host country sufficiently well for the purposes of communication in healthcare. According to Tomassini et al. (2022: 289), in their review of European legislation related to interpreting in healthcare settings, 'although detailed information is provided about how to obtain medical treatment in each Member State, the websites containing this information and leaflets for cross-border patients make no reference to concrete ways in which language barriers can be overcome.' In accounting for the different contexts of healthcare systems across the EU, Angelelli (2019: 35) similarly underlines,

> Although it is obvious that access to information is crucial for anyone to pursue healthcare assistance in a member state, none of the four documents constituting the EU framework explicitly refers to language provision for EU citizens or legal residents in that condition. In the absence of a clear EU legislative guidance, each member state has its own legislation and those vary considerably from one member state to another.

In countries like Spain and Italy, where healthcare competences and responsibilities are shared between the State and the Regions or Autonomous Communities, for many years there have been considerable organizational dissimilarities across the national territories. As such, it will be useful to offer a brief introduction to the healthcare systems in these countries and in Romania, before moving on to the comparative analysis of the interviews conducted in the three countries.

3.1. Spain

In Spain, while the Ministry of Health is responsible for proposing and executing the general government guidelines on health policies, the Autonomous Communities have their own healthcare services. Each Autonomous Community divides its healthcare services into two basic health areas: (1) primary care, which is provided in health centres, and (2) specialized care, which is mainly provided in hospitals covering different specialities. Apart from the public health system, people in Spain can choose to have additional private health insurance, allowing them to receive healthcare in private hospitals. In such cases, patients can choose where to receive healthcare. As Tomassini et al. (2022: 291) explain,

> although there is no specific legislation on the right to translation and interpreting in healthcare services, this right can be inferred from the Spanish Law 41/2002 on patients' autonomy, as it states that information and consent should be comprehensible and appropriate to the needs of the patients.

To give an example of how this translates into regional legislation, Regional Law 3/2009 for the Region of Murcia states that patients should be able to understand the information provided to them; in the case of foreign patients, therefore, this might imply the need for translation/interpreting. The organization of communication with patients who have limited proficiency in Spanish is assigned to the Autonomous Communities, which are responsible for including the strategies and solutions in their Strategic Plans related to social services and healthcare. More precisely, many Autonomous Communities sign agreements with external companies that provide interpreting services. That is, for instance, the case of Interpret Solutions, a company that offers telephone interpreting services for the social and healthcare services of several autonomous communities, adapting their services to regional needs.

As we will see in Section 4, some Spanish hospitals also have in-house interpreters or mediators; however, they are not directly hired by the hospital or health institution, but by the company that wins the tender, just like in many Italian regions, where the service is offered by local cooperatives. In both countries, though, the problem is that when language services are available, they are offered only in some facilities and at specific times of the day. Therefore, HCPs and HCUs cannot always benefit from such services, and at certain times and in some places fair access to healthcare by allophone patients is impossible in practice.

3.2. Italy

In Italy, as Bernardi and Gnani (2022: 56) argue, 'healthcare services are provided by regional governments', and therefore, significant differences are visible both in the services offered and in their overall quality. The European Observatory of Health Systems and Policies (<https://eurohealthobservatory.who.int/countries/italy>) confirms that,

> despite a strong commitment to equity in health care provision across regions, regional differences exist in population health status, access and quality of services. Northern and central regions generally have higher capacity and more advanced technology with care being perceived to be better quality, leading patients to travel to northern and central regions for services.

The current Italian National Health Service (*Sistema Sanitario Nazionale* or simply SSN) was created in December 1978 by Law no. 833. Inspired by the principles of universality, equality and equity, this law defines the facilities, services and activities needed to ensure the physical, mental and social well-being of the whole population, irrespective of individual and social conditions. A welfare system funded by national and regional taxes was created and organized in Local Health Authorities (*Aziende USL*), which since the 1990s have their own organizational, administrative, managerial and technical autonomy. A national system of quality and quantity control was also put in place and over recent decades, this monitoring system has been based on the assessment of Essential Levels of Care (*Livelli Essenziali di Assistenza* or LEAs), that is the 'national benefits package guaranteed to all citizens and registered foreign residents'.[1] LEAs are defined by the national Ministry of Health,[2] but it is the primary function of the Local Health Authorities to ensure that those levels are respected. More precisely, the regions independently plan and manage healthcare in the area under their jurisdiction, making use of both Local Health Authorities and university hospitals (*Aziende ospedaliero-universitarie*) where they are present. Since each Italian region has its own specificities – making it impossible to cover them all here – we will complete this short overview by providing one representative example of how public healthcare is deployed in regional, provincial and local bodies. For this we have chosen Emilia-Romagna because it is the Italian region with the highest level of foreign residents within the total population (Barbieri 2021: 28), implying that, by necessity, it has had to organize its healthcare services in such a way as to address the needs of foreign patients. In Emilia-Romagna, there are eight *Aziende USL*, which roughly correspond to its provincial territories, as well as four *Aziende ospedaliero-universitarie*, in the towns of Bologna, Ferrara, Modena and Parma. Each *Azienda USL* of the Emilia-Romagna region is then divided into Districts, and each District ensures the provision of services included in the LEAs to its target population. For example, the *Azienda USL della Romagna*, which is situated in the South-East of the region and covers the provinces of Forlì-Cesena and Rimini, has eight Districts and the Rimini District alone covers the needs of thirteen municipalities.[3]

---

1   See <https://eurohealthobservatory.who.int/countries/italy> where it is also specified that 'LEAs include hospital care, pharmaceuticals, outpatient health services, and rehabilitation and community health services. Over-the-counter pharmaceutical products are not covered and dental care coverage is very limited.'
2   The latest update on LEAs dates back to 2017, and a subsystem of 'core' indicators was also introduced in 2019.
3   For an overview of the organization of these services in the region, see <https://salute.regione.emilia-romagna.it/ssr/organizzazione/aziende-sanitarie-irccs/i-distretti-delle-aziende-usl>.

3.3. Romania

Similarly, the Romanian healthcare system also aims to ensure equitable and non-discriminatory access to a package of basic services for those covered by national health insurance. The country's National Health Insurance House (*Casa de Asigurări de Sănătate*, or CNAS) is an autonomous public institution, whose main object of activity is to ensure the uniform and coordinated functioning of the social health insurance system in Romania. According to the European Observatory on Health Systems and Policies (<https://eurohealthobservatory.who.int/countries/romania>),

> the Romanian social health insurance system (SHI) aims to provide universal health insurance coverage. In practice, SHI covered 89 per cent of the population in 2017. The state has a large presence in Romania's health system. The Ministry of Health is responsible for overall governance, while the National Health Insurance House (NHIH) administers and regulates the system.

At the local level, there are forty-two District Health Insurance Houses (*Casa Județeană de Asigurări de Sănătate*, or CJAS). Primary care is provided by family medicine physicians, under contract with the CJASs. As in Spain and Italy, in Romania there are university hospitals along with public or private hospitals, but the main difference, which will be illustrated more clearly in the comparative analysis below, is that there is no specific legislation ruling interpreting services, and thereby the access to healthcare services by foreign patients and refugees. Healthcare service providers who work with such users thus have to follow the provisions of various pieces of European and Romanian legislation (e.g. Law no. 272/2004 on Child Protection, Law no. 122/2006 on Asylum, and Law no. 292/2011 on Social Assistance), where the objectives of communication and non-discrimination are stated, but the means to reach them are not overtly explained.

4. Comparative analysis of results in Spain, Italy and Romania

This section presents a comparative analysis of the results obtained in the three countries and is organized into two main subsections: Healthcare providers' viewpoint (Section 4.1) and Healthcare users' viewpoint (Section 4.2).

4.1. Healthcare providers' viewpoint

The label *healthcare provider* (HCP) includes here a wide range of professionals who contribute, in some way or another, to providing healthcare services to native and foreign users in the three countries under scrutiny. Such professionals range from the heads of hospitals, health departments and clinics we interviewed in year 1 of the project, to the doctors, nurses, physiotherapists and care workers we interviewed in year 3. This provides us with a wide spectrum of viewpoints across the organizational structure of local healthcare facilities. Section 4.1 is further divided into five subsections, according to the topics discussed in the interviews, namely the legislative framework, the expectations concerning medical interpreting, the availability of language services, the pros and cons of ad hoc solutions and the providers' suggestions for improvement.

4.1.1. Legislative framework: From the letter of the law to local healthcare facilities

Given the specificities of the legislative and organizational scenarios in which the healthcare facilities of a specific country operate (see Section 3 and Angelelli 2019: 34–37), one could expect that the Spanish, Italian and Romanian HCPs would depict very different frameworks in the interviews. However, the comparative analysis of their answers showed similar issues being raised. To begin with, as Tomassini et al. (2022: 291) have already underlined in a chapter comparing legislation and opinions of top managers and associations in the three countries part of the study, 'there is no specific national legislation regulating medical interpreting, nor specific references to medical interpreters, in either national or regional legislation in any of the three countries involved in this study'.

SPAIN

On the issue of legislation, the Spanish interviewees talked about specific agreements made between local health authorities and external collaborators, such as associations of volunteer interpreters or interpreting companies. Only two of these interviewees referred to the legislation on the rights of patients. The provision of language services to foreign HCUs is, however, sometimes problematic 'as regards both the availability of interpreters and the failure of some companies to check on the training and qualifications of the interpreters they hire' (ibid.: 291–292). Consequently, although the letter of the Spanish law stipulates the right to healthcare, HCPs working in individual healthcare facilities are not always aware of the existing legislation. Their answers additionally show that such national and regional legislation does not always translate into adequate services at the local level.

ITALY

In the case of Italy,

> although there is no specific legislation regulating medical interpreting, the interviewees did, however, mention several documents, working groups and draft laws aimed at recognizing the profession of the cultural mediator, considered by interviewees to be far better than interpreters, who merely perform a 'linguistic translation', clearly revealing their lack of knowledge as regards the role of interpreters. (ibid.: 292)

Two important elements shall be retained from this quote, namely the proliferation of references to so-called intercultural mediators (*mediatori interculturali*) in Italian legislation and the confusion surrounding the professional figures of mediators and interpreters. We will briefly expand on the former, providing a short overview of recently introduced laws and standards in Italy, of which the interviewees could not be fully aware, while the issue of interpreters will be addressed in Section 4.1.2. As emerged from the interviews, in Italy there is still no national legislation on medical interpreters but there exist laws on intercultural mediators. This role was first mentioned in a law dating back to 1998 and then in a legislative decree of 2013 that aimed at creating a national system for the certification of competences. As interviewees stated, that decree remained stuck in Parliament for years, until a national framework of qualifications (*Quadro Nazionale delle Qualificazioni*) was finally established in 2018. As a consequence of the national legislative void, the Italian regions continued to act autonomously to establish the professional boundaries and curricular training of intercultural mediators. For the Emilia-Romagna region, Regional Council Resolution no. 936 (17 May 2004) establishes a system of qualifications, including that of intercultural mediator. This role is further described in Regional Council Resolution no. 1576 (30 July 2004), roughly establishing at 350–400 the number of intercultural mediators who should work not only for hospitals but also for social services, schools and courts in the region. Regional Council Resolution no. 2212 (10 November 2004) defines more precisely the intercultural mediator as a person who helps migrants to communicate with the relevant local authorities, removes language and cultural barriers, knows and promotes the migrants' culture of origin and helps them access private and public services. This Resolution thus places intercultural mediators in the professional area of social care, including them in a register of professional qualifications (*Repertorio delle professioni ISFOL*). Regional Council Resolution no. 141 (16 February 2009), introduced a few years later, describes the main competences of intercultural mediators and recommends specific training ranging from 300 to 500 hours in duration and including both formal education and practical experience. In parallel to the development of regional resolutions, Italian universities have created courses (see Chapter 2) on intercultural mediation, NGOs provide volunteer services, and a private not-for-profit association called UNI has developed a norm on professionals working in the field of translation and interpreting (UNI 11591:2015). In a significant achievement, this norm has recently been revised (UNI 11591:2022) and now clearly refers to the national framework of qualifications and to the UNI ISO 21998 standard on interpreting services in healthcare. However, HCPs and HCUs are generally not aware of this norm and continue to ask for intercultural mediators rather than interpreters, so the profession is not defined univocally across the country, and the two professions continue to work in parallel, alongside the ad hoc solutions that we will mention below.

ROMANIA

All Romanian interviewees admitted that there is no specific primary legislation governing medical interpreting in the country and stated that HCPs turn to several pieces of legislation that mention the right to non-discrimination, fair treatment and good communication. These three rights are also stated in the physicians' and nurses' national codes of ethics, where good communication means using terms that can be understood by the patient (Art. 10, Nurses' National Code of Ethics 2009), making sure the patient understands what is being communicated by the health professional and properly informing the patient before asking for informed consent (Art. 2, 11, 14, 27 the Code of Medical Ethics of Romanian College of Physicians 2016). These provisions are reinforced by Law no. 43/2003 on Patients' Rights (2003), in particular Article 8, which makes specific reference to language and states that information must be presented in clear and respectful language, and that, if healthcare users do not understand the official language, the information must be conveyed in a language they understand, either their native language or another.

In other words, the problem of interlinguistic communication is acknowledged in Romania, but, for the time being, no solutions are provided (unlike in the case of legal translators and interpreters, for which legislation does exist, although it is still not detailed enough). Along the same lines, we should mention that Article 25 of the Code of Medical Ethics of Romanian College of Physicians also refers to the importance of an 'unmediated relationship' between physicians and their patients.

It is also worth underlining that in Romanian law, interpreting is not distinguished from translation. As we will see in the next sub-section, the absence of such a vital distinction may explain a certain degree of confusion and misunderstanding that Romania shares with the other two European countries analysed here.

4.1.2. Varying levels of expectations concerning interpreting and mediation services

Starting from Tomassini et al.'s (2022: 297) conclusion that 'there is considerable ignorance as to the role of medical interpreters/cultural mediators' in the three countries under investigation, we will compare here the different expectations that were nonetheless expressed by the interviewees. Such expectations were discussed both in year 1, when the question was explicitly addressed to NGO representatives and to professionals at the top of the organizational structure, as well as in year 3, when some expectations emerged from the interviews with healthcare professionals interacting with foreign patients.

SPAIN

HCPs appeared to hold little awareness of the roles and duties of medical interpreters. Interviewees mentioned the key principles of confidentiality and data protection and generally stated that the main function of interpreters is that of *translating*, thereby showing a similar misunderstanding to that found in Romania over the terms *to translate* and *to interpret* as they understand *interpreting* as something else than '*just translate*', going further than when translating. Just like their Romanian counterparts, some Spanish interviewees consider that the interpreter should translate but not interpret. This opinion is visibly in contrast to what Seleskovitch and Lederer (2001) state in their pioneering work *Interpréter pour traduire*, whose title implies that one cannot translate without interpreting, in its first meaning of making sense of what participants are saying before rendering it into another language. Interestingly, however, greater awareness came from one Spanish NGO representative, who highlighted the importance of the interpreter's cultural competence, as problems in the communication might arise that are more related to culture than to language.

ITALY

In this country, interviewees had much clearer expectations of the people ensuring communication with allophone patients, although their answers revealed a similar lack of understanding of what *interpreting* implies. When talking about their expectations in this area, most of the interviewees referred to intercultural mediators, and according to the representative of one NGO, the ability to mediate conflicts should be one of the two competences of mediators, alongside a socio-pedagogical competence that would be visible when they actively listen to patients and welcome them. Similar to what emerged in Spain, the two Italian NGO representatives underlined in their interviews that language and culture are both crucial in helping patients and their families to access healthcare services, and privacy and neutrality were also considered key indicators of service quality. Italian heads of hospitals and health departments were even more precise in stating their expectations. In their view, intercultural mediators must be trained and experienced, in other words, they need to hold exact and in-depth knowledge of what participants may discuss in a specific health context. They also stated that intercultural mediators must be willing to engage in dialogue between HCPs and HCUs in both oral and written forms, and therefore rapport building and the translation of medical forms are also expected of them. Finally, Italian interviewees see language as part of a wider framework of expectations, which one of them clearly linked to five different levels of intervention in the provision of intercultural mediation services:

1. the 'psychological and relational' level, which aims at assessing the needs and resources of immigrant service users;
2. the 'educational and informational' level, which relates to the orientation of relations between immigrant service users and service providers and includes training on access to services, the organization of services, and related procedures and regulations, so that intercultural mediators can then provide foreign patients with such information;

3. the 'cultural' level, which helps ensure the understanding of the cultural codes of all parties involved in communication between HCPs and foreign HCUs, and aims at improving the knowledge of specific groups of patients in managing illness and health;
4. the 'linguistic and communicative' level, which refers to the provision of oral and written translation with the aim of helping providers better understand what immigrant service users need;
5. the 'organizational' level, which aims at orienting the services by designing guidelines, actions and new services in line with immigrant or ethnic minority service users' needs.

In short, according to Italian interviewees, interpreters would cover only part of these goals and expectations, while intercultural mediators would cater for a wider range of needs. In their view, whenever doctor-patient communication occurs, it is always mediation that is required, while in situations where Italian doctors are talking to foreign doctors, interpreting is required, implying that mediation is used in asymmetric interactions, while interpreting is used in symmetric interactions (on asymmetries in the medical setting see Lázaro Gutiérrez 2013). However, such a distinction clearly does not match current understandings of the role of the interpreter: in the UNI revised norm mentioned in Section 3, the knowledge of interactional dynamics and potential asymmetries is in fact one of the distinctive features of medical interpreters, and medical interpreting requires specific skills that are listed in the norm. Interestingly, however, no interviewee mentioned this norm, which uses the term *mediation* not to describe the different levels of intervention of intercultural mediators but rather to cover the whole range of professional activities of translators and interpreters. Even more interestingly, while providers at the top of the organizational structure always used the term *mediator* to talk about the person ensuring communication with foreign patients, providers working directly in the field also used the term *interpreter*. This was especially the case for a nurse and a doctor working in two different facilities of the Emilia-Romagna region, who clearly stated the advantages and disadvantages of different solutions and made practical suggestions to improve interpreting services, which will be further discussed in Section 4.1.5.

ROMANIA

In line with its legislation, interviewees often made no distinction between *translating* and *interpreting*, but all seemed to hold clear expectations of those who ensure communication with allophone patients. Based on their knowledge of the communication requirements for the talk-based medical profession, as well as on their experience with ad hoc interpreters (see Angelelli 2019: 29 for a definition), they mentioned several required competences. Three of these stand out as most important in their view; namely accuracy (one interviewee, head of a hospital department, said that the patient's words should not be *interpreted*, but rendered with no trace of subjectivity), confidentiality and the knowledge of medical terminology. Romanian interviewees also mentioned communication skills, neutrality, familiarity with the Romanian healthcare system and, in one case, the mastery of both languages, including their various registers and dialects.

4.1.3. From individual solutions to organized language services: The spectrum of responses across the three countries

Our three-year research project confirmed the initial findings by Tomassini et al. (2022: 293) that 'there is no standard approach to resolving language barriers in any of the three countries and that healthcare institutions frequently resort to ad hoc solutions'. Starting from this common premise, we can, however, make some distinctions between the exclusively individual solutions adopted in Romania and the tentatively common services that exist in Spain and in Italy, where the decentralization of services and the different funding allocated by each region partly explain the absence of a fully nationwide solution and the existence of scattered pilot experiences.

SPAIN

The decentralization of services partly explains the lack of a unitary solution in Spain, where hospitals at least try to create their own common resources, thereby providing healthcare professionals with a range of possibilities to overcome linguistic and cultural barriers. The most widely used are relatives, friends and members of the same linguistic community, followed by healthcare professionals working in the facility who know foreign languages, and then by organized volunteers and interpreters – be they professionals working on site or for remote interpreting companies that win a tender for offering their services for a number of years. Local healthcare facilities additionally resort to pictograms adapted to different languages and cultures, as well as to translated documents. However, interviewees said that only a small number of documents are translated – usually documents such as informed consent forms – and then only into the most common languages, such as English, French and Arabic. Some interviewees even told us that they had translated some documents themselves and one provided us with a webpage created by the Spanish Association of Paediatric Emergency Doctors containing documents translated into different languages. Almost all interviewees admitted to using automatic translation services such as Google Translate, not only for written documents but also for oral communication with patients who cannot read. Some interviewees said that they worked with external translation and interpreting companies for some languages and usually for fixed times in the day. However, they underlined that it is impossible to have interpreters at every moment, and when they are not available, providers either resort to ad hoc interpreters provided by the patients themselves or try to speak in a foreign language they know (some studied English or French in school), making use of gestures and drawings when needed. Interestingly, they added that when they use a foreign language, their intention is not to translate 'properly' but to make the patient understand at least some information, and they also acknowledge that this is not always a good solution because their command of the foreign language is not sufficient. Some interviewees also complained that whenever they do not have an interpreter, they have to keep the information to a minimum, that is, they try to present the most important elements but do not cover all the issues they would raise with Spanish-speaking patients, which has clear implications in terms of fair and equal access to healthcare.

From the interviews conducted in Spain, we can thus conclude that there is not a homogeneous provision of services, since even though all the interviewed healthcare professionals were working in public hospitals across the country, they answered differently depending on the facility. Even within the same region, answers were very different if the interviewee was working in the main hospital or elsewhere. From their answers, we can, however, infer that the language combinations available in the interpreting services do not meet the existing needs, and when patients speak a different language, they are advised to bring their own interpreter. In the event that patients come on their own, people in the waiting room may be used as interpreters; this is recognized as a problematic solution but is sometimes the only option available. Some Spanish healthcare professionals also referred to problems with Ukrainian patients, probably due to the fact that most interviews were conducted after the Russia-Ukraine war began in February 2022. However, it is important to note that there was already a high number of Ukrainians living in Spain before the war. What is more, it is unclear whether the limited number of language combinations used in Spanish healthcare facilities is because other languages are not offered by face-to-face translation/interpreting companies, or simply because providers are not aware of the outsourced interpreting services available. The crucial point here is that even in hospitals where interpreting *is* provided, not all professionals are aware of the existence of this service, and they often learn about it only by chance (a similar situation can be seen in Italy, as will be discussed below). Once HCPs start using interpreting services, some complain that the system is not straightforward and that, for example, in the emergency department, they cannot use the service because they have to book it in advance, which is clearly not possible in emergency cases. It is worth specifying that all the information gathered in Spain was related to hospitals, as we had no interviewees working in public health clinics. None of the HCPs interviewed worked for private hospitals, but according to the data gathered in year 2 of our research (see Chapter 2 in this volume), some private hospitals hire in-house interpreters, usually according to the language combinations needed. However, English again tends to be used as a *lingua franca* for patients whose languages are not common in the country, so the language coverage is not sufficient to meet the needs of all foreign patients and ensure them fair access to Spanish healthcare.

ITALY

Just like in Spain, in Italy there is no nationwide solution to language and cultural barriers, but attempts made by the Local Health Authorities for their various Districts and facilities can roughly be divided into two categories: so-called 'linguistic and cultural mediation services' deployed in hospitals as well as in routine local services such as family counselling on the one hand, and ad hoc solutions on the other. Mediation services are generally offered by intercultural mediators (and sometimes interpreters) working for the cooperative that wins a tender for a certain number of years and guarantees availability at certain times of the day. These mediators generally live in the area and are familiar with the facilities within that specific Local Health Authority, which according to interviewees is a significant advantage, since it enables them to offer far more than 'mere' linguistic mediation, thereby achieving the expected educational and informational goal stated in Section 4.1.2. Interviewees stated that, when available, such services work well: providers are confident that the messages are rendered correctly (two recurring words in the interviews were 'ease' and 'certainty'), and as far as they can tell, the patients seem happy with the service. In the HCPs' view, remote forms of interpreting can also be useful if it is 'just a matter of' linguistic mediation, with video being preferred rather than telephone interpreting because it is considered more human than just a voice (see Angelelli 2019: 31 on the use of video 'that emulates most closely the in-person experience'). However, HCPs interviewed in year 3 raised two problematic issues which may partly explain the reason why doctors (and patients, as we will see) are not always aware of the existing services (similar to the case of Spain) and why professionals resort to some of the individual solutions we will also find in Romania. Providers firstly mentioned the paucity of interpreters/mediators for large institutions with many foreign patients, and secondly they lamented the time it takes to activate the service, which is often not provided when needed (again, very similar to the situation in Spain). Italian HCPs consequently argued that many healthcare professionals prefer not to call interpreters/mediators (some additional reasons for this will emerge in Section 4.1.4), and they also stressed the absence of any reference to interpreting/mediation services in university courses, which explains why Italian providers often get to know the service by chance (unsurprisingly, this is very similar to their Spanish counterparts). In light of all these limitations, Italian healthcare units and/or their individual hospitals also resort to non-professional solutions, which were mentioned not only by NGO representatives and heads of hospitals/health departments in year 1, but also by healthcare staff interviewed in year 3. This includes solutions that are also used by Romanian and Spanish providers, such as relatives and friends onsite or over the phone, volunteers, web apps and the use of *linguae francae*, especially English and French, which appear to be widely used in the three European countries within this study. Italian interviewees additionally mentioned child language brokering, Italian language courses for migrants, as well as the use of non-verbal forms of communication such as gestures, which are also resorted to whenever the mediation service is unavailable.

Summing up the Italian situation, when the number of interpreters/mediators is sufficient, the service is timely, and the language combinations offered are adequate to local needs, there appear to be some good examples of services that are both available and well appreciated. That is, for instance, the case of the *Azienda USL della Romagna*, where, in hospitals located in a touristic area along the Adriatic coast, English, French and German are needed and offered. However, providers agreed that this is not the case at all times and in all places, and they also stressed that not all members of the healthcare staff speak English sufficiently well for the special purposes of communication in healthcare, which hinders their direct communication with patients. In the regions of Emilia-Romagna, Lombardy and Piedmont, where most of the interviewees came from, interpretation/mediation services generally cover French, German, Russian and Arabic in addition to English. However, many other languages are not sufficiently covered by the available services. According to our interviewees, this is the case for Albanian, Chinese and for Slavic languages other than Russian, such as Bosnian/Croatian/Serbian, Czech, Polish and, last but not least, Ukrainian, for which in Italy, just like in Spain, ad hoc solutions are often the only ones possible.

ROMANIA

Medical interpreting is not a distinct profession in the Romanian classification of occupations and, consequently, it is not regulated as such. According to the interviews with HCPs and also those with experts, decision makers and representatives of NGOs and associations, each healthcare facility has a list of options they tend to favour. Individual solutions are found for each situation, depending mainly on the language combination needed. Whenever possible, certified translators/interpreters are used, but being a certified interpreter does not imply that one is indeed trained or specialized in healthcare interpreting. To make things worse, in the case of refugees who speak languages or dialects that are not taught in Romania, certified interpreters are not a viable solution, unless the patients also speak a *lingua franca*, generally English or French. Interpreters are sometimes contacted through consulates or embassies and, in their absence, nurses or auxiliary medical staff may provide interpretation or translation. In the region of Transylvania, it is not uncommon for medical staff to speak Hungarian, so they can assist patients who are better able to express themselves in this language. Social workers or other employees of NGOs or of the healthcare institution may also act as interpreters, thereby fulfilling two roles at a time: interpreter *and* professional in their respective fields, with all the advantages and disadvantages we will review below. Sometimes doctors and patients have one common language and two scenarios can be identified: either both speak English (usually as a foreign language) or both speak a common language (usually their mother tongue) – in Romania this is most often Hungarian, but there are also doctors whose mother tongue is Turkish (from the Turkish community in the Dobrogea region) or Arabic (graduates of Romanian universities who originate from Arabic-speaking countries). Interestingly, as two interviewees pointed out, doctors may even be selected for employment at the hospital on the basis of the languages they speak. Finally, family members or acquaintances may also act as ad hoc interpreters. In the case of refugees, a common solution is that of relying on another refugee who has been in Romania for a longer period of time and who speaks a little Romanian in addition to the language or dialect of the person who requires interpretation. Additionally, help can be provided by members of the respective ethnic communities. This list of solutions was confirmed by the interviews with doctors, as well as through the workshops conducted with medical professionals in year 3. We can thus confirm the initial results of Tomassini et al. (2022: 294), who stated that 'in Romania there is no single strategy, nor any kind of coordination of efforts between healthcare providers', who are thus left to find individual solutions to the specific communication issues that arise.

4.1.4. Pros and cons of using ad hoc solutions from HCPs' perspectives

HCPs also commented on the pros and cons of ad hoc solutions, especially on the use of family members and healthcare staff. Spanish and Italian providers, on the one hand, had generally tried both language professionals and ad hoc solutions, and were thus in the position to take stock and to mention some differences and implications we will briefly recall below, first accounting for results or year 1 (representatives of healthcare institutions and departments) and then of year 3 (healthcare professionals). HCPs interviewed in Romania, on the other hand, seemed well aware of the risks of ad hoc solutions and interpreters, but had never worked with specialized medical interpreters – given that such a specialization does not exist in their country – so it was understandably hard for them to make proper comparisons and this is why Romania is not covered here.

The Spanish representatives of healthcare institutions mainly mentioned the following points:

- unlike professional interpreters, ad hoc interpreters can be selective in what they interpret and may not have a good enough understanding of Spanish to accurately interpret;

- unlike professional interpreters, ad hoc interpreters do not usually know specialized terminology;
- when using family members and friends as ad hoc interpreters, the privacy of the patient is compromised (problems were reported when the interpreter was the patient's husband).

While acknowledging these differences and being aware that, when using ad hoc interpreters, providers need to analyse the information carefully without relying too much on what has been translated, some interviewees still did not see the need for professional medical interpreters. In their view, language barriers can be overcome with alternative strategies, and some even said that cultural barriers can be far more problematic than linguistic ones. The cultural element was also stressed by Italian interviewees, especially by the heads of departments and healthcare services interviewed in year 1. In their opinion, interpreters are technical experts who can translate information for patients literally, thus ensuring the first two points above, but who lack the necessary cultural background to enable patients to fully understand the situation, its gravity and the implications of certain conditions. Mediators, on the other hand, are perceived as professionals trained to facilitate communication in healthcare settings where language is not the only variable and where people belonging to the same ethnic group are believed to better understand patients' expectations and cultural presuppositions (on the risk of different presuppositions and expectations between HCPs and HCUs, see Baraldi et al. 2012 and Angelelli 2019). In addition to mediators, relatives and friends are also considered extremely important, since they can help create a 'bridge' and a bond between healthcare service users and providers, thereby contributing to socio-emotional communication and the forging of relationships.

In both Spain and Italy, the healthcare professionals interviewed in year 3 showed different degrees of awareness compared to interviewees in year 1. Spanish HCPs were relatively unaware of the pros and cons of using family members as interpreters and some considered that, since these people know the patient better, they are better placed to provide doctors with more information. In their view, family members concentrate not only on information transmission but also on the transfer of feelings, which only partially compensates their lack of fluency in Spanish and their lack of knowledge of medical terminology. They also stated that children are sometimes used as interpreters, and while they believe that this is not an ideal solution, they also state that it is sometimes the only option available. Spanish healthcare professionals seem happy when their colleagues act as interpreters, since they consider them to have sufficient medical knowledge, which appears to be the most important issue for Spanish HCPs.

Greater awareness of the ad hoc solutions and their (dis)advantages was found among the Italian HCPs interviewed in year 3. When admitting that they resorted to Google Translate and other automatic translation applications, they underlined that they did not trust these apps, because they cannot check the accuracy of the translations. A nurse also said that even when professionals know English – or German in some rarer cases – they use medical jargon. While this is sufficient to communicate with peers, like other doctors in a conference, it is not enough to talk to patients, who generally do not understand medical terminology but speak about their illnesses and symptoms in lay terms, with the 'voice of the lifeworld' (Mishler 1984). Italian healthcare professionals also expanded on the pros and cons of using family members and colleagues to interpret. In the case of family members, they believe that the cons outweigh the pros. Although relatives generally accompany the patient and are thus easily available upon the patient's arrival,[4] they may not be available outside visiting hours or when they work, which is a problem if the patient is admitted to a ward. Italian professionals additionally lamented the possibility of dominant partners speaking for the patient (husbands were mentioned in Italy just like in Spain), or of children lacking an understanding of medical procedures and terminology. Inaccuracy or incompleteness in an interpretation may not only be linked to a lack of understanding, which can happen with children and adults alike, but also to the withholding of information (or 'gatekeeping') when it comes, for example, to the delivery of bad news, or as a result of shame, anxiety and taboos, which may prevent the family

---

4   This was not the case during the COVID-19 pandemic, when family members had no or very limited access to the facility if the patient was elderly.

member from rendering all that is said by a participant. As for the use of colleagues working in the same healthcare facility, in the view of HCPs, the pros here outweigh the cons, because, although this means that they stop doing their job and thus cause a disservice to their own department while interpreting (see the dual-role mentioned by Romanian interviewees above as well as by Angelelli 2019: 5), they are generally more easily accessible and available for longer periods of time. What is more, colleagues know medical procedures and forms (interviewees reported that they are often called for the signing of informed consent forms), they speak the same medical language as the provider (which confirms the importance of medical knowledge that Spanish professionals also underlined), and they can correctly 'interpret' and render the message for the patient, thereby also facilitating rapport building. A nurse working in the Emilia-Romagna region interestingly told us that professionals always need to *interpret* what the patients are saying, even when there are no linguistic barriers, which reminded us of Angelelli's (2019: 47, our emphasis) words about providers who 'are trained in listening and in *interpreting* what patients are trying to say'. In the nurse's view, doing such interpretation with a patient who speaks another language is – in her words – an interpretation of an interpretation, which can be 'different' and 'deeper' if it is a colleague who is helping to communicate with the foreign patient.

4.1.5. Healthcare providers' suggestions for improvement

HCPs in general, and doctors and nurses in particular, see interpreting and mediation services through their own professional lenses, which appears to have both advantages and drawbacks. On the negative side, the fact that their opinions are based on what happens in their own professional field makes it hard for them to distinguish professional from unprofessional interpreters. This issue clearly emerged from interviews conducted in Spain, where healthcare professionals tend not to be aware of whether the interpreter is really a professional interpreter, or even if they have any training at all. They tend to think that, since this person has been sent by the translation/interpreting company, s/he has the required training to provide interpreting. Unfortunately, however, this is not always the case, as some companies do not check the background and experience of their interpreters, nor do they provide them with training. It is important to note here that interpreting, and particularly medical interpreting, is not a regulated profession, which means that in Spain, but also in Italy and Romania, 'anyone who knows two languages' can interpret. To perform as a healthcare professional, on the other hand, one has to demonstrate the requisite skills and training to carry out the tasks of the profession. Therefore, healthcare professionals tend to think that the same applies to interpreting, and that if a person has been sent as an interpreter, s/he is a professional.

On the positive side, the fact that HCPs see interpreting services from the point of view of their own profession enables them to provide useful suggestions that language and communication professionals may not envisage. This is an issue that clearly emerged from two interviews conducted with an Italian nurse and an Italian doctor working in two different hospitals of the *Azienda USL Romagna*, in the Emilia-Romagna region. To begin with, both insisted on the need to institutionalize and better structure the available interpreting/mediation services, which in their view can be done in different ways. Their basic suggestion is to make a clear distinction between time-dependent situations/contexts and those requiring longer admission to specific units, in other words, between the demands of the emergency department and those of other hospital wards where patients have a range of changing needs over longer periods of time. On the basis of this crucial distinction – and of one other important distinction between cases where remote interpreting can be effective and those where it is not – one could work to improve services in the two contexts. As for the emergency department, the interviewed doctor underlined the importance of having an interpreter accompany the patient all the way from admission in triage through to the different consultations/exams. Based on this doctor's experience, such an interpreter can act as a crucial link between different healthcare units and professionals, which is what already happens in some emergency services of the Emilia-Romagna region.[5] Not only in

---

5   For instance, in the hospital where this doctor used to work, qualified interpreters give voice to possible changes in patients' feelings and narrative, from the moment

the emergency department but also in other units where doctors deal with particularly sensitive issues (e.g. reproductive health), the availability of gender-concordant interpreters is seen as an important improvement to be made. One interviewee, a nurse on an emergency surgery ward, thus suggested that the concept of on-call availability generally associated with healthcare professionals be extended to include language professionals, be they interpreters or mediators. To improve other types of healthcare units, where patients may stay even longer, the same nurse also suggested that routine interpreters'/mediators' visits be organized (e.g. ten-minute visits scheduled on a regular basis in each ward that regularly receives foreign patients). By doing so, the ward staff would know when language professionals are coming, and they could optimize their service, that is, by concentrating the linguistic and cultural issues of different patients and/or by anticipating possible communication issues that may arise depending on the evolution of the patient's condition. In her view, this is what already happens with certain healthcare professionals, for example, with physiatrists who are not permanently in the surgery ward but come regularly to assess specific aspects of patients' conditions. Therefore, in the view of this interviewee, there is nothing to prevent this good medical practice from being transferred to language services. According to both the doctor and the nurse, context-specific demands can be anticipated in training, but internships in healthcare facilities are crucial for would-be interpreters to see what their experienced colleagues are saying and doing, which was also suggested by interviewees in year 1. To acquire the needed experience interpreters should – as one interviewee said – 'steal with their eyes' from experienced professionals, in the same way healthcare professionals do through compulsory internships during their university years. Healthcare professionals, on

---

they first talk with nurses at triage, to the time when they first address the doctor. The entire process could potentially take a number of hours, if the emergency department is crowded and the condition is not life threatening, so the fact that interpreters can see and report those changes is, in the interviewee's view, highly valuable. In the doctor's opinion, this may imply something different from what is generally stated in interpreters' codes of ethics, given that interpreters are not only translating what primary participants are currently saying but also relaying what has been said before, in the triage.

the other hand, should participate in joint interprofessional training with interpreters, so that they become familiar with interpreting/mediation services at university and learn to work with them before the need arises. Finally, for those HCPs who do not speak English sufficiently well for the purposes of communication in healthcare – the vast majority, according to our Italian interviewees – organizing courses in English for Specific Purposes (ESP) is also paramount for improving access to healthcare services by foreign language users.

4.2 Healthcare users' viewpoint

When analysing the quality of interpreting services, studies tend to concentrate on the perspectives and opinions of professionals. It is important to highlight that HCUs' views have to be considered because they are the *recipients* of the healthcare services (Angelelli 2019). However, contrary to what many professionals tend to think (i.e. that it is the users who require the interpreting service), interpreting services are needed equally by both parties: without interpreting, healthcare professionals face greater difficulties in performing their job and allophone patients do not receive nor perceive the same quality of treatment as national patients.

This section, in which the results of the interviews with HCUs carried out in the three countries are presented, is divided into four subsections according to the major topics that emerged in the interviews.

4.2.1. Availability of professional interpreting services in healthcare settings

According to HCUs from the three countries, patients do not have access to interpreting services, a situation which appears to be systemic because even where interpreting or mediation services *are* available, they are not necessarily used and patients are not informed of their existence. This is in line with what we have seen in previous sections: too often healthcare professionals are not sufficiently aware of this service. In HCUs' view, the absence of interpreting services in healthcare facilities is in line with what happens in other public institutions, where they also have to communicate without any language support. HCUs state that they cannot count on HCPs (doctors, nurses, administrative staff at helpdesks) speaking English, nor on the forms to be read and completed being translated into a language they understand. In the case of the HCUs interviewed in Spain, they had never had the possibility of using a professional interpreter, in general relying on an ad hoc interpreter – usually a relative or friend or simply someone who happened to be at the hospital at the time interpretation was needed but who was not a trained interpreter. These people who had needed an interpreter when arriving to the country acted as ad hoc interpreters themselves after becoming fluent in Spanish, and often after having experienced the lack of such a professional. The most similar experience to having a professional interpreter was reported by one interviewee who was helped by a bilingual HCP who was able to speak English.

Patients indicate that, in their experience, there is usually no information in languages other than the country's official language and that forms are only available in the official language, with a few exceptions (in some hospitals, forms are available in English or French). In this respect, while patients do not expect to have forms and information in their native language, they expect them to at least be available in English or French as a *lingua franca*.

SPAIN

In the case of the interviews conducted in Spain, only the two interviewees who spoke English (either as their native language or as a *lingua franca*) indicated that at times they were able to communicate directly with some HCPs in a language other than Spanish, but that this was not the case every time they needed assistance. According to the interviewees, the availability of someone speaking other languages depends mostly on the people who are working at the healthcare facilities at any given time, and not on the type of healthcare facility (healthcare clinic, hospital, emergency department, etc.). Even English-speaking patients are asked to bring their own interpreter, with some healthcare facilities displaying handwritten posters asking patients to bring their own interpreter. For other languages, as we will present in the following section, patients need to resort to their own solutions to communicate with healthcare staff.

ITALY

As for the language combinations offered, the interviews carried out in Italy revealed that patients consider that the language combinations available often depend on local needs and communities, without any systematic organization at a national level. HCUs agree with HCPs on the fact that healthcare staff does not speak English sufficiently well for the special purposes of communication in healthcare. The other foreign languages that are generally covered in addition to English are Russian and Croatian, mainly during summer months, while languages such as Arabic, Albanian, Chinese and other Slavic languages such as Bosnian/Croatian/Serbian, Czech, Polish and Ukrainian are not sufficiently covered by the available services, because, as patients report, only Russian is taught at universities in the country. HCUs disagree with HCPs on the issue of Arabic language provision, with HCUs finding that the language is not sufficiently covered, while HCPs believe it is.

ROMANIA

The situation in Romania is similar to that in Spain. According to the interviewees, it is very difficult to communicate in healthcare settings unless the HCU speaks Romanian, English or French. However, speaking French or English does not guarantee successful communication either, as many healthcare professionals do not speak these languages.

4.2.2. Solutions adopted to eliminate linguistic barriers

The results obtained from a qualitative analysis of the interviews conducted in year 3 showed similar results for the three countries participating in the project. All interviewees stated that, before being able to speak the language of the host country, when they needed someone to communicate with healthcare staff, they usually relied on a friend or relative. Some of the interviewees later became ad hoc interpreters themselves for family members and extended family and would also interpret for friends who had just arrived in the country. Some had in fact already acted as interpreters when they were children. One of the HCUs interviewed in Spain told us that she had acted as an interpreter for her family and that this experience was behind her decision to pursue a Degree in Translation and Interpreting, so that she could help others avoid going through what she went through as a child. Even in the cases where they do not work as interpreters on a regular basis, many of the interviewees who once were allophone patients have worked as ad hoc interpreters for other users. Interviewees stated that when the visit to the healthcare facility was not to an emergency service, they would attend accompanied by someone who can help them to understand the language. The accompanying person then translates the doctor-patient dialogue and mediates any cultural issues (related to food, religion, etc.) that may arise during the communication.

HCUs interviewed in Italy mentioned some of the ad hoc solutions found, namely the use of family members or friends who know both Italian and the foreign language and the use of partners (e.g. one's girlfriend) along with the use of *linguae francae*, mostly in cases where the patient and the professional can speak some English, or French in fewer cases.

Some interviewees consider the use of children as interpreters to be normal practice. However, others state that the use of children is usually restricted to situations with the family doctor, where they felt the issues dealt with were easier than those addressed by other specialized doctors. For these more specialized doctors, patients stated that they try to attend the appointment accompanied by a friend or relative. Children who act as interpreters do so not only for their parents but also for other relatives and friends. Studies on the consequences of using children as interpreters have mainly focused on the United States (Antonini and Torresi 2021), and research findings remain inconclusive; while some children might like to interpret in such situations as it gives them a sense of pride for helping their families, others see interpreting as a huge responsibility that puts them under pressure and causes them to worry about not doing the work sufficiently well (Weisskirch and Alatorre Alva 2002; Bauer 2012).

In the case of Romania, one of the main solutions mentioned by HCUs – mostly for Hungarian patients and probably due to the immigration and historical context – was the use of bilingual staff, that is, Hungarian or Hungarian-speaking nurses, who help to interpret or speak directly in Hungarian to the patient. Other HCUs in Romania again reported that patients usually go to the hospital linguistically prepared, that is, they bring a relative or a friend to help them to communicate. It is also interesting to mention that, according to the interviewees, in the private healthcare system in Romania written documents, such as informed consent forms, are translated into a language other than the official one, mostly English or French.

One solution mentioned in the three countries by HCPs but not by HCUs is the use of machine translation applications to communicate in healthcare settings. This is probably because this solution is not widespread in healthcare services, possibly because most of the time HCUs are accompanied by someone speaking the official language and thus do not need to resort to this means.

From the interviews it seems that patients are generally satisfied with healthcare services despite the communication difficulties they might encounter. One explanation for this is that patients are happy that they are able to receive treatment for their health issues and are not fully aware of the beneficial consequences of having a qualified interpreter to help them with communication. Another reason might be that, since most of the time they bring their own ad hoc interpreter, they do not really feel the need for a professional interpreter, as long as they are able to communicate their problem to the doctor.

4.2.3. Healthcare users' experiences when using ad hoc interpreters

Experiences when using ad hoc interpreters are varied and seem to depend on the results of the consultation. It is interesting to note that most of the interviewees, who had once needed interpreting services, later went on to act as interpreters themselves after learning the official language of the country. Interviewees therefore also spoke about their own experiences as interpreters. As we have mentioned before, and at least in the case of Spain, most of the interviewees were once recipients of interpreting carried out by a friend (when they first arrived and they did not speak the language), but as soon as they were able to express themselves in the official language, they themselves became ad hoc interpreters for others. One of the interviewees stated that being an interpreter as a child put a great deal of pressure on her, because she and her brother did not know the terminology and were afraid of making a mistake when interpreting for their parents. In the case of Italy, a foreign (female, Ukrainian) patient working as a caregiver reported on her experience of ad hoc interpreting for a Russian lady who was in Italy to visit her daughter; she had been taken to hospital by ambulance but did not understand why, and doctors were unable to communicate with her. The interviewee explained that the lady's daughter had accompanied her mother but could not speak Italian at all, and that she was the only person able to ensure communication with the medical staff. Her report clearly shows that on that occasion, several years ago, no communication was possible between healthcare professionals and this elderly Russian patient in that hospital, which could have led to a real emergency, as the doctors were unable to obtain any information from the patient. Only after running some tests, it turned out that, fortunately, it was simply a case of high blood pressure and that the patient had no significant health problems. However, had the health condition been more serious and had the interviewed HCU not been at the hospital at that time, there would have been an impenetrable linguistic barrier that could have led to significant consequences for the patient.

As far as the use of partners for language mediation is concerned, one of the HCUs interviewed in Italy expanded further on his experience when his girlfriend – who would usually interpret for him – was not available. He provided two useful insights into the advantage of using professional intercultural mediators instead of ad hoc solutions when explaining medical problems to the service providers, be they doctors or staff at help and reception desks. Firstly, since the mediator was able to clearly communicate the problems and obstacles, he felt much more secure because he had passed the communicative responsibility on to the mediator and secondly, he was able to explain everything in his own language without feeling the need to invent words, find shortcuts or draw on a piece of paper. Having said this, the same Serbian patient admits that he managed to communicate with doctors and staff at helpdesks directly and explained that when the interpreter was not available, he used English as a *lingua franca*.

Some other interviewees also mentioned using English as a *lingua franca* for communication when the HCU and HCP speak a shared language other than the language of the host country, often English, which is then used by the HCP to speak directly to the patient without the need for any third party. One interviewee in Italy stated that some doctors hold a positive bias towards native English speakers and that this enabled her, as a native English speaker, to receive better treatment when communicating directly with them. She also indicated that the times she had to speak in Italian to high-level medical professionals, the fact that she did not know the words in Italian but did know them in English always worked to her benefit, because even though it was clear that she had an accent when speaking in Italian and that she could not speak the language well, they managed to understand her. However, she considered that there was a huge difference in the treatment received by her, as a native speaker of English, and that received by other immigrants speaking other languages.

There are other cases in Spain and Romania when the effort made by HCPs to speak to HCUs in English is mainly seen in a positive way. In Spain, this was the case for a native English-speaking patient and for a Polish patient who could communicate in English and German.

Some interviewees reported bad experiences when using ad hoc interpreters. One Romanian patient interviewed in Spain reported that on one occasion her mother went to the hospital on her own; she did not speak any Spanish and therefore, as none of the HCPs could speak Romanian, the hospital staff called on someone working in the kitchen. This person interpreted incorrectly and changed the meaning (saying that the woman was allergic to medication that was important for her treatment). The problem was not solved until the woman visited the doctor accompanied by her Spanish-speaking daughter, after which she received the correct treatment and her condition improved.

Sometimes, the lack of an interpreter can lead to significant problems, as one of the interviewees in Romania, a HCU from Morocco, reported. In this case, the HCU had contracted COVID-19 during the pandemic and needed to call an ambulance. At that point in time, the HCU spoke Romanian at A2 level and was not proficient enough to fully communicate his situation, while the triage nurses spoke neither English nor French. Although the nurses followed protocol, the HCU had an allergy to a medication he was given, and, as a result of the treatment, had to be admitted to hospital. After this, he called the Honorary Consul of France in Cluj and the Consul himself had to interpret.

4.2.4. Healthcare users' suggestions for improvement

According to most interviewees, there is a need to offer more interpreting services and also to better inform both HCUs and HCPs of their existence. Interviewees also commented that more information about the service should be made available, for example, through posters displayed in the waiting rooms in the most encountered languages. However, it is important to bear in mind that the system works as follows: HCPs are the ones who should contact the interpreters in the first place if they realize that there might be communication problems in the three countries.

In Spain, suggestions for improvement are related to the ability of HCPs to speak a *lingua franca*, such as English or French, at the triage stage, as a means of ensuring at least minimal communication. While this is not an ideal situation either, if the patient speaks that language, it is considered an adequate way to overcome communication issues at the initial admission stage. Similarly, some interviewees consider it important that ambulance drivers speak English so they can communicate when they pick up a patient. Some users also agreed with the use of remote interpreting as a way of improving communication for allophone patients and healthcare professionals. However, they also indicated that they had never used such a service.

In the case of Italy, HCUs considered that interpreters and mediators should be able to speak several languages, at least in main/regional hospitals. Two interviewees considered that interpreting services should be institutionalized, with one arguing that the only way such a service could really work was if interpreters were part of the institution and the planning process, thus ensuring that the services offered through interpreters are co-created with the interpreters themselves. This same HCU, a native English speaker, also added an interesting point about written materials, which she later formulated as a direct suggestion for the improvement of written documentation used in healthcare facilities. She stated that everything in the hospitals *was* in English but was mostly incomprehensible, that most of the written materials had not been written directly in English but translated from Italian and did not make much sense to her. She believed that if these documents were difficult to understand for a native speaker of English, someone using English as a *lingua franca* would probably not be able to understand them.

A male Serbian HCU interviewed in Italy also suggested the institutionalization of interpreting services, based on two separate experiences he had in the Emilia-Romagna and Trentino regions. In his opinion, there should be a methodical procedure when a foreign patient who does not speak the country's official language arrives at the hospital: an interpreter should be automatically requested and the patient would therefore feel more relaxed, knowing that there would be someone to support him/her in communicating his/her issues.

A third HCU interviewed in Italy presented an amalgamation of the suggestions of the two previous interviewees, suggesting an improvement in the language of forms, the institutionalization of services and the filtering of allophone patients; this interviewee stated that the most basic suggestion would be to complete forms before someone attends the actual medical appointment to determine the patient's linguistic needs.

One of the interviewees from Romania reflected on the idea of confidentiality when using ad hoc interpreters, even if they are healthcare professionals or students and the importance it should have in the course of interpreting. Finally, but of no less importance, this interviewee indicated that having professional interpreters would reduce stress, not only for patients, but also for healthcare professionals.

6. Conclusions

As stated by Angelelli (2019: 22), 'hospitals, clinics and community health centres are organizations embedded in specific societies'. In this chapter, we have tried to account for how Spanish, Italian and Romanian healthcare organizations are embedded in their respective countries on the basis of information gathered from people on the front line, that is, healthcare service providers and users. After introducing our methodology in Section 2, in Section 3 we provided a short overview of the healthcare systems and legislation in Spain, Italy and Romania. Section 4 was then organized into two main subsections, one giving voice to HCPs and the other to HCUs. From the comparative analysis of their viewpoints, which we will briefly recall below, we can conclude that Spain, Italy and Romania are at different stages of their development, which we will summarize borrowing on Schuster's (2013) model of language access to public institutions.

This five-stage sociological model describes and analyses the processes leading from a chaotic public sphere in which no institutionalized and professional solutions are in place to facilitate communication between service providers and members of a linguistic minority, to a public sphere that is linguistically accessible as part of a comprehensive policy of cultural competence. The model proposed by Schuster (2013: 63) includes the forces impacting the process, such as those that facilitate or hinder full language access. The following are the stages of the model:

A. Chaos
B. Emerging awareness
C. Piloting professional interpreting services
D. The decisive phase:
   D1. Disappearance of the service
   D2. Small-scale projects continued
   D3. Expansion, Duplication and Institutionalization
E. Spillover

HCUs interviewed in the three countries were not as precise as HCPs in talking about solutions adopted to eliminate cultural and linguistic barriers, instead they simply state that interpreting services do not exist. In the case of Spain, users seem to take for granted that they need to attend medical appointments with someone who speaks the country's official language, and that it is normal to bring one's own ad hoc interpreter, because they appear to assume that it is their duty to take responsibility for enabling communication with HCPs. Users thus forget that interpreting services are necessary for both sides: the interpreter is needed by HCPs to provide quality healthcare and by HCUs to receive the correct treatment. In any case, HCUs were surprised to learn that interpreting services do exist in some hospitals.

In Italy, users substantially agreed – among each other and with providers – on the need to institutionalize interpreting services to ensure that they are linguistically appropriate, sufficient in availability, and timely. Their suggestions for improvement are based on personal (often negative) experiences and take two main directions: better translations of written documents, which could be used to filter allophone patients from the moment they access the healthcare facility; and linguistic assistance and guidance throughout the path of care, starting from the moment in which patients' linguistic needs have been determined and appropriate interpreters are methodically assigned.

As for Romania, it seems that at least sharing a *lingua franca* with the HCPs would satisfy the HCUs, but the fact remains that the situation is extremely chaotic in the countries under investigation and that if we only considered the beliefs of the users interviewed, the three countries would probably be at stage A of their development according to Schuster's (ibid.) model.

If we consider the HCPs' viewpoints, however, some differences emerge between the three countries. In the case of Romania, while it is true that 'the state does not provide comprehensive and institutional means of linguistic access' (ibid.: 63) and that 'the service provider must resort to ad hoc solutions' (ibid.) – two typical conditions of the chaos A stage – it is also true that interviewees showed an emerging awareness. According to Schuster (2013: 64), awareness is generally the result of different processes and forces, such as scientific research and the knowledge of solutions adopted in other countries, to which ReACTMe undoubtedly contributed. We may thus conclude that, at least partially thanks to this three-year Erasmus+ project, Romania is currently moving from the stage of chaos (A) to that of emerging awareness (B), although some obstacles still prevent it from piloting professional interpreting services and thus from moving to the third (C) stage of development. In the words of Schuster (2013: 66),

> Stage 3 of the model entails the founding of a designated professional interpreting service, usually for a trial period. This service may be part of an organisation or public service, or may be an independent (profit- or non-profit) organisation that subcontracts interpreting services to public institutions.

This quote recalls the system of subcontracts with companies, associations and cooperatives that we have found both in Spain and Italy, through which, according to HCPs, some interpreting and mediation services are available. However, despite some commendable pilot attempts, most of the services are insufficient in number, language provision and timeliness; there is thus a need for further research and partnerships for these two countries to face the decisive stage of their development. To quote again Schuster (2013: 67), who draws inspiration from the ground-breaking volume *The Critical Link: Interpreters in the Community* (Carr et al. 1997),

> Partnerships with members of academia who deal with interpreting are important in ensuring a professional and reliable service based on proven models and on standards of ethical practice. Researchers can assess needs, perform quality control, and evaluate performance, thereby helping to create strategic plans for the future of language access.

To conclude, we may say that both Spain and Italy are in the fourth decisive (D) stage of their development, where following Schuster (2013: 67) there are three main options for proceeding: (D1) the disappearance of the few services available and the return to a state of chaos; (D2) the continuation of a small-scale operation of the service, which implies that many regions and local health authorities will go on adopting ad hoc solutions, with the advantages and disadvantages listed above; or (D3) the expansion, duplication and institutionalization of the good services that currently exist.

This third direction entails not only the introduction of the successful interpreting services described by our interviewees into additional institutions, but also the introduction of national legislation and regulations ensuring that interpreting is included in the regular budget. Although we can hardly impact on the latter, we do hope that the ReACTMe project has made a contribution to mapping what exists and what is still lacking in Spain, Italy and Romania in terms of medical interpreting, thereby providing commendable examples and useful suggestions for exiting the current 'limbo stage' between chaos and full access (ibid.: 69) and to improve the healthcare and language services nationally and Europe-wide.

Bibliography

Angelelli, Claudia. 2019. *Healthcare Interpreting Explained*. London: Routledge.
Antonini, Rachele, and Ira Torresi. 2021. 'Child language brokering in healthcare settings', in Şebnem Susam-Saraeva and Eva Spišiaková (eds), *The Routledge Handbook of Translation and Health*. London: Routledge, 471–476.
Baraldi, Claudio, Federico Farini, and Laura Gavioli. 2012. 'La mediazione sanitaria e la visibilità del paziente (migrante)', in Claudio Baraldi (ed.), *Gli invisibili: La condizione degli immigrati nella società*. Acireale-Roma: Bonanno Editore, 149–176.
Barbieri, Marzio. 2021. *La mediazione inter-culturale in Emilia-Romagna: Uno strumento per le politiche di inclusione e contrasto alle disuguaglianze*. Bologna. <https://sociale.regione.emilia-romagna.it/documentazione/pubblicazioni/prodotti-editoriali/2021/la-mediazione-inter-culturale-in-emilia-romagna-uno-strumento-per-le-politiche-di-inclusione-e-di-contrasto-alle-disuguaglianze>.
Bauer, Elaine. 2012. 'Reconstructing moral identities in memories of childhood language brokering experiences', *International Migration* 51(5), 205–218.
Bernardi, Eleonora, and Francesca Gnani. 2022. 'The impact of the COVID-19 pandemic on medical interpreters/cultural mediators in Italy', *FITISPOS International Journal* 9(1), 54–77.
Codul de etică și deontologie al asistentului medical generalist, al moașei și al asistentului medical din România [Nurses' National Code of Ethics, Art. 10,

16, 21, 27]. 2009. <https://legislatie.just.ro/Public/DetaliiDocumentAfis/ 236239>.

Garwood, Christopher, Almudena Nevado Llopis, Ana Isabel Foulquié Rubio, Elena Tomassini, Alina Pelea, Alina Andreica. 2023. 'Ethical dilemmas in medical interpreting – helping trainee interpreters decide', in Julian Bourne, María Manuela Fernández Sánchez, Juncal Gutérrez Arcacho, Tatiana Portnova Macarena Pradas Macías, Enrique Quero Gervilla (eds), *Reflexiones sobre ética profesional de traductores e intérpretes y buenas practices Nuevos contextos en la profesión y en la formación*. Granada: Comares, 163–182.

Gerolimich, Sarah. 2015. 'Introduction', in Sara Vecchiato, Sonia Gerolimich, and Nickolas Komninos (eds), *Plurilingualism in Healthcare: An Insight from Italy*. London: BICA, 23–30.

Giarelli, Guido. 2008. 'Il contesto della mediazione: La sfida dell'interculturalità nella società multietnica', in Claudio Baraldi, Viola Barbieri, and Guido Giarelli (eds), *Immigrazione, mediazione culturale e salute*. Bologna: FrancoAngeli, 15–45.

Hsieh, Elaine. 2006. 'Conflicts in how interpreters manage their roles in provider-patient interactions', *Social Science & Medicine* 62(3), 721–730. <https://doi.org/10.1016/j.socscimed.2005.06.029>.

Lege nr. 122 din 4 mai 2006 (*actualizată*) privind azilul în România [Law no. 122/2006 on Asylum in Romania, 2006]. <http://legislatie.just.ro/Public/DetaliiDocument/71808>.

Lege nr. 272 din 21 iunie 2004, Republicată privind protecția și promovarea drepturilor copilului [Law no. 272/2004 on the Protection and Promotion of the Rights of the Child, 2004]. <www.mmuncii.ro/j33/images/Documente/Legislatie/L272-2004-R.pdf>.

Lege nr. 292/2011 din 20 decembrie 2011, Legea asistenței sociale [Law no. 292/2011 on Social Assistance, 2011]. <https://mmuncii.ro/j33/images/Documente/Legislatie/Assistenta-sociala-2018/Legea_asistentei_sociale_18012018.pdf>.

Legea drepturilor pacientului, Monitorul Oficial Nr. 51 din 29 ianuarie 2003 [Law no. 43/2003 on Patients' Rights, 2003]. <https://legislatie.just.ro/Public/DetaliiDocumentAfis/41483>.

Lázaro Gutiérrez, Raquel. 2013. 'Natural interpreters' performance in the medical setting', in Christina Schäffner, Krzysztof Kredens, and Yvonne Fowler (eds), *Interpreting in a Changing Landscape*. Amsterdam: John Benjamins, 165–185.

Leanza, Yvan. 2005. 'Roles of community interpreters in pediatrics as seen by interpreters, physicians and researchers', *Interpreting. Journal of Research and Practice in Interpreting* 7(2), 167–192.

Ley 14/1986, de 25 de abril, General de Sanidad [Law 14/1986 of 25 April, General Health]. <www.boe.es/buscar/act.php?id=BOE-A-1986-10499>.

Ley 16/2003, de 28 de mayo, de cohesión y calidad del Sistema Nacional de Salud [Law 16/2003 of 28 May on the Cohesion and Quality of the National Health System].

Mishler, Elliot G. 1984. *The Discourse of Medicine: Dialectics of Medical Interviews*. Norwood, NJ: Ablex.

Ozolins, Uldis. 2000. 'Communication needs and interpreting in multilingual settings: The international spectrum of response', in Silvana E. Carr, Roda P. Roberts, Aideen Dufour, and Diana Abraham (eds), *The Critical Link 2: Interpreters in the Community. Selected Papers from the Second International Conference on Interpreting in Legal, Health and Social Service Settings*. Amsterdam: John Benjamins, 21–33.

Regional Council Resolution No. 141. (2009), Approvazione di nuove qualifiche professionali, ai sensi della del. G.R. n. 2166/2005 e modifiche agli standard professionali e formativi della qualifica per 'Mediatore interculturale', di cui alle del. G.R. 2212/2004 e 265/2005, Deliberazione della Giunta Regionale Emilia Romagna 16 febbraio. <https://bur.regione.emilia-romagna.it/archivio/inserzione?anno=2009&prog_documento=1&num_boll=46>.

Regional Council Resolution No. 936 (2004), Orientamenti, metodologia e struttura per la definizione del Sistema Regionale delle Qualifiche, Deliberazione della Giunta Regionale Emilia Romagna 17 maggio. <http://bancadati.italialavoro.it/bdds/ViewScheda.action?product=NORMALAVORO&uid=0fdeb187-09a2-4e01-a25a-8200904a4b74&title=scheda#>.

Regional Council Resolution No. 1576 (2004), Prime disposizioni inerenti la figura professionale del 'Mediatore interculturale', Deliberazione della Giunta Regionale Emilia Romagna 30 luglio. <https://bur.regione.emilia-romagna.it/archivio/inserzione?anno=2004&prog_documento=2&num_boll=152>.

Regional Council Resolution No. 2212 (2004), Approvazione delle qualifiche professionali in attuazione dell'art. 32, comma 1, lettera c, della l.r. 30 giugno 2003, n. 12 – 1° provvedimento, Deliberazione della Giunta Regionale Emilia Romagna 10 Novembre. <http://bancadati.italialavoro.it/bdds/ViewScheda.action?product=NORMALAVORO&uid=95ae3d59-9271-4509-b7ab-28cae2e4b3dc&title=scheda>.

Regional Law 3/2009 of 11 May on the rights and obligations of healthcare system users in the Region of Murcia, Ley 3/2009, de 11 de mayo, de los derechos y deberes de los usuarios del sistema sanitario de la Región de Murcia. <www.boe.es/buscar/pdf/2011/BOE-A-2011-2493-consolidado.pdf>.

The Romanian College of Physicians (RCP), Code of Medical Ethics of the Romanian College of Physicians, Art. 2, 11, 14, 25, 27, (2016), Printed in Monitorul Oficial (Official Journal), Part I No. 981, from 7 December 2016. <https://esamis.org/uploads/pdf/Code-of-Medical-Ethics.pdf>.

Royal Decree-Law 7/2018 on Universal Access to the National Health System, Real Decreto-ley 7/2018, de 27 de julio, sobre el acceso universal al Sistema Nacional de Salud. <www.boe.es/buscar/doc.php?id=BOE-A-2018-10752>.

Schuster, Michal. 2013. 'From chaos to cultural competence: Analyzing language access to public institutions', in Christina Schäffner, Krzysztof Kredens, and Yvonne Fowler (eds), *Interpreting in a Changing Landscape*. Amsterdam: John Benjamins, 61–82.

Seleskovitch, Danica, and Marianne Lederer. 2001. *Interpréter pour traduire*. Paris: Didier.

Sleptsova, Marina, Gertrud Hofer, Eggler Marcel, Paul Grossman, Naser Morina, Matthis Schick, Mary-Louise Daly, Irina Weber, Oktay Kocagöncü, and Wolf Axel Langewitz. 2015. 'What do interpreters understand as their role in a medical consultation and how do they carry it out in reality?', *Psychotherapie, Psychosomatik, Medizinische Psychologie* 65(9–10), 363–369. <https://doi.org/10.1055/s-0035-1554691>.

Tomassini, Elena, Almudena Nevado Llopis, Ana Isabel Foulquié Rubio, Mette Rudvin, Alina Andreica, and Alina Pelea. 2022. 'Medical interpreting in Spain, Italy and Romania: A comparative study', in Maria Pilar Castillo Bernal and Marta Estévez Grossi (eds), *Translation, Mediation and Accessibility for Linguistic Minorities*. Berlin: Frank & Time, 287–301.

UNI 11591. 2015. *Attività professionali non regolamentate – Figure professionali operanti nel capo della traduzione e dell'interpretazione*. <https://store.uni.com/uni-11591-2015>.

UNI 11591. 2022. *Attività professionali non regolamentate – Figure professionali operanti nel capo della traduzione e dell'interpretazione*. <https://store.uni.com/uni-11591-20022>.

UNI ISO 21998. 2021. *Servizi di Interpretariato – Interpretariato in ambito sanitario – Requisiti e raccomandazioni*. <https://store.uni.com/p/UNI1609581/uni-iso-219982021-310383/UNI1609581_EEN>.

Vecchiato, Sonia. 2015. 'Introduction', in Sara Vecchiato, Sonia Gerolimich, and Nickolas Komninos (eds), *Plurilingualism in Healthcare: An Insight from Italy*. London: BICA, 11–20.

Weisskirch, Rober S., and Sylvia Alatorre Alva. 2002. 'AlvaLanguage brokering and the acculturation of Latino children', *Hispanic Journal of Behavioral Sciences* 24, 369–378. <https://doi.org/10.1177/0739986302024003007>.

ALMUDENA NEVADO LLOPIS, FRANCESCA GNANI AND
ALINA PELEA

2 Medical Interpreter Training in Spain, Italy and Romania: State of Affairs and Expectations for the Future

1. Introduction

Training is one of the primary elements to be considered when pursuing the professionalization of medical interpreting. For this reason, year 2 of the ReACTMe project (2020–2021) was dedicated to a comparative analysis of formal training in medical interpreting in the three participating countries: Spain, Italy and Romania. With this objective in mind, the existing literature on medical interpreting training was reviewed. Afterwards, a detailed study of university-level translation and interpreting programmes and their curricula was conducted and focus groups with higher education representatives as well as translation and interpreting trainers and professional medical interpreters were held. Non-university training for medical interpreters also exists in Spain and Italy, but this falls outside the scope of our present research, and therefore will not be analysed in detail in this chapter.

Involving universities, key players in interpreter training, in our research, allowed us to obtain empirical information with respect to the situation in the field and, at the same time, to make contact with those who are the most likely to benefit from and contribute to the implementation of the extracurricular module on medical interpreting developed as part of the ReACTMe project, which is described in Chapter 6 of this volume.

2. Methodology

The comparative analysis was conducted using different ways of collecting data. Firstly, the websites of the Spanish, Italian and Romanian universities offering training in interpreting were examined with the aim of obtaining an overview of the curricula of their translation and interpreting degrees, and to discover how many medical interpreting courses, or courses in related fields, they offered. In analysing the websites, we looked for the following data for the courses offered: number of ECTS, type of course (elective or compulsory), language combinations and general information about methodology and learning outcomes.

However, before arriving at the analysis of the curricula, a document analysis of various different sources was needed to determine the existing university-level programmes on translation and interpreting in the three countries.

In the case of Spain, a number of different online tools were employed, such as QUEDU (*Qué Estudiar y Dónde en la Universidad* [What to Study and Where at University]), created by the Ministry of Education, Culture and Sport (MECD); Universia, an open network that brings together more than eight hundred associated universities in twenty countries (Fundación Universia); and Educaweb (<www.educaweb.com>), a private educational website for academic and professional guidance. Additionally, various official documents published by the Spanish Ministry of Education, the Spanish Register for Universities, Centres and Degrees (RUCT) and the General Technical Secretariat of the Ministry of Universities (SGTMU) in Spain were consulted. Moreover, a literature review of books and papers dealing with translation and interpreting training was conducted. Finally, data provided by the Spanish Office for National Statistics (INE) was also essential in allowing us to determine the number and origin of migrants and tourists coming to Spain and then compare these data with the languages studied within translation and interpreting degree programmes offered in the country.

In Italy, a mapping of the existing bachelor's and master's degrees was carried out through an online search of university-level degrees in

Translation and Interpreting Studies as well as in Intercultural Mediation in all twenty Italian regions. Universitaly, the website of the Italian Ministry of Education and Research (MIUR), which offers information on existing courses, was also consulted to scan all L12 (code identifying bachelor's courses on language mediation in Italy) and LM94 (code identifying master's courses on interpreting and translation in Italy) courses.[1] To assess whether the language combinations offered by these courses meet market needs, the 2019 Italian National Institute of Statistics (Istat, <www.istat.it>) census of the migrant population residing in Italy was consulted and the current flow of tourists was broken down by nationality.

To gain an overview of interpreter training in Romania, the analysis started from the lists of accredited bachelor's (BA) and master's (MA) degree programmes for the 2021–2022 academic year published by ARACIS, the Romanian Agency for Quality Assurance in Higher Education (Guvernul României 2022a, 2022b, 2022c). From these lists, degree programmes that included training in interpreting, specialized translation and/or intercultural communication were selected, and their individual curricula, obtained from the departmental websites or through communication with programme directors, were analysed. Elements considered during the analysis were the existence or absence of courses in medical interpreting, public service interpreting, consecutive interpreting, simultaneous interpreting, specialized translation, medical translation and terminology. At this stage, the place of such courses in the overall context of each degree (i.e. whether several types of interpreting and interpreting modes are combined, whether interpreting and translation

---

[1] There are also a number of non-university courses offered by associations/cooperatives in collaboration with local or regional bodies. Such organizations award the 'Intercultural Mediator' Vocational Training Certificate or qualification, which is legally valid (Law 845/78 and Regional Council Resolution 129, 22/02/2016) in Italy and EU member states. The duration of these courses varies from 120 to 330 class hours and from 150 to 200 hours of on-the-job experience. Courses are often aimed at mediators working for immigration departments, local offices, schools, hospitals, courts and prisons, cooperatives and associations promoting sociocultural integration projects. Since such courses lie outside the scope of this research, a detailed description will not be presented in these pages.

run in parallel within one degree) and the description of the graduates' professional profile were also taken into consideration. The search for a scientific and documented analysis of interpreting studies in Romania yielded no results, so the present ReACTMe research might be the only recent endeavour in this direction. The data from the document analysis was, finally, compared with the immigration figures for Romania (Eurostat 2022) to see if the linguistic needs are met by the training programmes in interpreting.

The second way of collecting data, as already mentioned in the introduction, consisted of the organisation of focus groups, held with professional (medical) interpreters, interpreter trainers and policy decision makers in higher education in the three countries under study. The main objective of these focus groups was to understand the perspective of professional interpreters and trainers working in the sector in Spain, Italy and Romania regarding the current situation of medical interpreting, training needs, best practices and expectations. The questions asked to the first group, made up of professional interpreters, were the following:

- What is your relationship with the institution where you work?
- Is there any difference between a conference/business/legal interpreter and a medical interpreter?
- Do you think that medical interpreters need specialized training?
- What competences (knowledge, skills, attitudes) do you think a medical interpreter should have?
- If you have ever performed medical interpreting, did you follow specific ethical guidelines?
- If you have ever performed medical interpreting, do you think that healthcare professionals and foreign-language-speaking patients understood your role?

For the second group, made up of trainers and higher education representatives, the questions posed were as follows:

- Are medical interpreting courses offered by Spanish/Italian/Romanian universities?

- What language combinations are offered by Spanish/Italian/Romanian translation and interpreting degrees?
- Do you think that these language combinations answer the linguistic and cultural needs in Spanish/Italian/Romanian healthcare services?
- Is there any difference between a conference/business/legal interpreter and a medical interpreter?
- Do you think that medical interpreters need specialized training?
- What competences (knowledge, skills, attitudes) do you think a medical interpreter should have?
- What kind of training methods and resources would you use for training medical interpreters?

The focus groups were organized remotely using videoconferencing tools (specifically, Zoom and Microsoft Teams); with the participants' permission, the sessions were recorded and then transcribed verbatim to facilitate the data analysis.

3. Comparative analysis

3.1. University medical interpreting courses

3.1.1. Spain

According to the analysis conducted in Spain, close to 40 per cent of Spanish universities (that is, thirty-one out of eighty-three) offer programmes in Translation & Interpreting Studies, specifically, thirty-one BA and twenty-six MA programmes. Within those degree programmes, there are twenty courses on medical interpreting or related fields[2] which

---

2   The total number of courses offered is slightly higher if one considers the courses with different language combinations (as in the case of UJI and UGR) as separate courses.

are mainly offered at postgraduate level or in the final years (third and fourth years) of the BA programmes, as can be seen in Table 2.1:

Table 2.1. Courses related to medical interpreting offered at Spanish universities

University	Degree	Name of course	Year[3]
Universidad Autónoma de Barcelona (UAB)	MA in Translation and Intercultural Studies	Introduction to Public Service Interpreting	
		Settings in Public Service Interpreting	
		Practices in Public Service Interpreting	
Universidad de Alcalá (UAH)	MA in Intercultural Communication and Translation and Interpreting in Public Settings	Healthcare Interpreting	
Universidad de Alicante (UA)	BA in Translation and Interpretation	Interpreting	3
Universidad de Granada (UGR)	BA in Translation and Interpretation	Introduction to Public Service Interpreting B/C-A	4
Universidad de Las Palmas de Gran Canaria (ULPGC)	MA in Professional Translation and Intercultural Mediation	Liaison Interpreting	

3 The year in which the courses are studied is only mentioned in the case of the BA programmes, since all the MA programmes included in the table have a one-year duration.

Table 2.1. Continued

University	Degree	Name of course	Year[3]
		Interpreting and Mediation in Public Services	
		Note-taking for Intercultural Mediation	
Universidad de Murcia (UM)	BA in Translation and Interpretation	Public Service Interpreting B-A	4
Universidad de Valladolid (uVa)	BA in Translation and Interpretation	Social Interpreting	4
Universidad de Vigo (UVIGO)	BA in Translation and Interpretation	Liaison Interpreting	3
Universidad Pablo de Olavide (UPO)	MA in International Communication, Translation and Interpreting	Social Interpreting	
Universidad San Jorge (USJ)	BA in Translation and Interpretation	Public Service Interpreting	4
		Intercultural Mediation	3
Universitat Jaume I (UJI)	BA in Translation and Interpretation	Intercultural Mediation and Interpretation A1 – B/B – A1 in Public Service Domains	4
	MA in Medical and Healthcare Translation	Mediation in Healthcare Settings	
		Interpreting Techniques for Healthcare Settings	
	MA in Research in Translation and Interpretation	Methodology of Research in Intercultural Mediation and Translation in Healthcare Settings	

(*continued*)

Table 2.1.   Continued

University	Degree	Name of course	Year[3]
		Mediation and Translation in Healthcare Settings	
Universitat de Vic (uVic) and Universitat Oberta de Catalunya (UOC)	BA in Translation, Interpretation and Applied Languages	Teleinterpretation	4

As already stated in previous research on interpreter training in Spain (Martin 2015; Camacho Sánchez 2019; Álvaro Aranda and Lázaro Gutiérrez 2021; Nevado Llopis and Foulquié Rubio 2023), the great majority of these courses (sixteen out of twenty) are elective and they have between 3 and 6 ECTS credits. It is worth noting that training in medical interpreting is mostly included in more general interpreting courses or in courses with a broader scope (such as public service interpreting courses – which also deal with interpreting in other settings, such as legal interpreting or police interpreting – or intercultural mediation courses), and in some cases, dealing with the healthcare setting in such courses depends on the trainers' own interests and experience.

Concerning the languages studied in these programmes, as can be seen in Table 2.2, English and French are the most frequent B languages offered, with the exceptions of UAB, UAH, UA and UGR, which also offer other B languages within their programmes: Chinese (UAB and UAH), German (UA and UGR) and Arabic (UAH and UGR). This means that the language combinations that are mostly studied within Translation and Interpreting degree programmes in Spain are generally Spanish-English or Spanish-French (very few universities offer combinations with other languages, such as German and Arabic and, to a lesser extent, Chinese and Russian or other European languages, mainly Italian and Portuguese – and these mainly as C languages).

Table 2.2. Languages studied within degree programmes in translation and interpreting in Spain

University	Degree	B language/s	C language/s	D language/s[4]
Universidad Autónoma de Barcelona (UAB)	MA in Translation and Intercultural Studies	Chinese English		
Universidad de Alcalá (UAH)	MA in Intercultural Communication and Translation and Interpreting in Public Settings	Arabic Chinese English French Russian		
Universidad de Alicante (UA)	BA in Translation and Interpretation	English French German	English French German	Arabic Chinese Italian Polish Romanian Russian Greek
Universidad de Granada (UGR)	BA in Translation and Interpretation	Arabic English French German	Arabic Chinese English French German Greek Italian Portuguese Russian	
Universidad de Las Palmas de Gran Canaria (ULPGC)	MA in Professional Translation and Intercultural Mediation	English		

(*continued*)

[4] By 'D language' we understand the third foreign language studied in a translation and interpreting degree programme to which less study time is devoted.

Table 2.2. Continued

University	Degree	B language/s	C language/s	D language/s[4]
Universidad de Murcia (UM)	BA in Translation and Interpretation	English French	Arabic English French German Italian	
Universidad de Valladolid (uVa)	BA in Translation and Interpretation	English	English French German	
Universidad de Vigo (UVIGO)	BA in Translation and Interpretation	English French	English French German Portuguese	
Universidad Pablo de Olavide (UPO)	MA in International Communication, Translation and Interpreting	English		
Universidad San Jorge (USJ)	BA in Translation and Interpretation	English	French	
Universitat Jaume I (UJI)	BA in Translation and Interpretation	English	German French	
	MA in Medical and Healthcare Translation	English		
	MA in Research in Translation and Interpretation	English		
Universitat de Vic (Uvic) and Universitat Oberta de Catalunya (UOC)	BA in Translation, Interpretation and Applied Languages	English	French German	

One can conclude that this offer of language combinations only partially meets the language needs of the Spanish healthcare services. The offer matches the nationality of tourists visiting Spain, who, according to the data collected over the last year by INE, the Spanish National Institute of

Statistics, mainly come from the United Kingdom, France and Germany (INE 2022b), and therefore presumably speak English, French and German. However, the offer does not correspond to the mother tongue of the largest allophone immigrant communities living in the country, who, according to the data provided by INE, shown in Table 2.3, are from Morocco, followed by Romania, and then the United Kingdom, Italy, China, Germany, France and, to a lesser degree, Bulgaria, Portugal and Ukraine:

Table 2.3. Country of origin of the fifteen largest foreign communities living in Spain

Country of origin	Number of residents
Morocco	776,223
Romania	632,859
United Kingdom	316,529
Colombia	315,885
Italy	298,817
Venezuela	220,461
China	193,129
Germany	143,079
France	128,050
Honduras	125,435
Ecuador	121,113
Peru	118,299
Bulgaria	117,056
Portugal	107,326
Ukraine	105,760

Source: INE (2022a: 3)

The learning outcomes found in the syllabi of the studied courses can be classified as follows: acquisition and development of general competences (such as the ability to reflect, critical thinking, the ability to identify and solve problems or the capacity to work autonomously and in teams) and acquisition and development of more specific competences (such as linguistic and (inter)cultural competence or the ability to interpret in consecutive and simultaneous mode and to perform sight translation). However, thematic competence (understood, as explained in Chapters 4 and 6 of this volume, as knowledge of the context in which the interpreter works) is scarcely mentioned, especially as far as knowledge about how healthcare services work or about the different procedures and documents used in these contexts is concerned. This is not surprising given that very few courses focus exclusively on medical interpreting, with the majority related to interpreting in general, public service interpreting or intercultural mediation.

Finally, according to the analysed syllabi, the methods employed in the university courses related to medical interpreting in Spain are mainly practical, based on cooperative and problem-solving learning, with little attention given to theory. Exercises mentioned in the syllabi include pre-interpreting exercises (analysis and synthesis, memory, rephrasing, etc.) and interpreting exercises (simultaneous interpreting, consecutive interpreting and note-taking, liaison interpreting, sight translation). Based on the information provided in some methodology sections of the studied syllabi, role plays are frequently used and are sometimes recorded for their subsequent analysis.

To summarize, while some courses related to medical interpreting can be found in Spanish universities, specific courses with the duration and language combinations required to meet the needs of healthcare services are scarce. Exceptions can be found in the MA in Medical and Healthcare Translation offered by UJI, with two courses (8 ECTS in total) specifically related to interpreting and mediation in healthcare settings, but only with the language combination English–Spanish, and the MA in Intercultural Communication and Translation and Interpreting in Public Settings offered by UAH, with one healthcare interpreting course (5 ECTS) which, according to the information published on the university's website, offers a range of language combinations, including Arabic, Chinese, French, English and Russian.

3.1.2. Italy

According to the analysis carried out in Italy, there are many degree programmes offered in interpreting and translation or cultural/intercultural mediation by universities or SSMLs (*Scuole Superiori di Mediatori Linguistici*, Linguistic Mediation Schools), under different names. According to the *Universitaly* database of the Ministry of Education and Research (MIUR), there are 34 BA programmes on Cultural Mediation (L12) and 14 MA programmes in Translation and Interpreting (LM94) offered at universities throughout the country, as well as 54 SSLMs offering undergraduate degrees in Translation and Interpreting, making a total of 102 degree programmes throughout Italy.[5] None of these programmes offer courses that are specifically devoted to medical interpreting, even though medical interpreting is taught in several dialogue interpreting courses as part of a wider learning programme and in several cultural mediation courses. In addition, some medical interpreting courses are offered by universities as advanced training courses (*Alta Formazione*).

In L12 BA programmes, the topics and courses offered are mainly of a general nature (foreign languages, linguistic mediation, translation, sight translation, IT skills, linguistics and theoretical subjects, soft skills), but some universities have also introduced modules on dialogue interpreting in the healthcare setting. Unfortunately, much depends on the personal initiatives and experience of trainers. For example, at the Università di Bologna – Campus di Forlì (UNIBO-Forlì), trainers in dialogue interpreting decided to teach a business module in the second year and a healthcare or legal module in the third year, while one trainer on this course focused on breast cancer for three consecutive years. At Università degli Studi Internazionali

---

5   In 1999, a university reform was passed in Italy and the former 4/5-year-degree programmes were replaced by 3-year BAs, and 2-year MAs (which can be accessed only after being awarded a BA). For the purposes of our research, we took into consideration the L12 BAs (degrees in Cultural Mediation), the LM94 MAs (degrees in Translation and Interpreting) and the SSLMs (*Scuole Superiori di Mediatori Linguistici*, Linguistic Mediation Schools) which are institutes awarding an undergraduate degree according to the Ministerial decree no. 38 dated 2002; such a degree is considered equivalent to those awarded by standard universities.

di Roma (UNINT), in the third year there is a module introducing medical interpreting within the wider English language course. The English course taught on the BA in Applied Interlinguistic Communication at the Università degli Studi di Trieste (UniTS) includes a module on simulated dialogue interpreting in the healthcare sector. Medical interpreting is also taught in the dialogue interpreting course (language combination Italian-German and Italian-Spanish) of the BA in Linguistic and Intercultural Mediation at the Università degli Studi G. d'Annunzio Chieti – Pescara (Ud'A). Finally, at the Libera Università di Lingue e Comunicazione (IULM) the healthcare sector is among the subjects of the dialogue interpreting course taught in all three years.

In LM94 MA programmes, the subjects taught are more specific, such as dialogue interpreting, consecutive and simultaneous interpreting, etc. In some Translation and Interpreting faculties, medical interpreting is taught within courses on dialogue interpreting, even though, once again, this is left to the discretion and experience of trainers. At UNINT, for example, ten years ago, a group of trainers teaching dialogue interpreting autonomously decided to split the course into three sections: business, medical and legal settings. The course was then modified three years ago, since when trainers have officially taught only business liaison interpreting. UNIBO-Forlì has a course in the theory and praxis of specialized dialogue interpreting that deals with complex interactions in the medical field and other sectors. In general, medical interpreting is not easily found in MA course syllabi but is generically mentioned in the general description of the objectives of the overall degree programmes.

As touched upon above, besides universities there are also SSLMs that mention medical interpreting in the descriptions of their degree courses; however, specific information about the content covered is hard to find. To mention just a few examples, SSML Gregorio VII in Rome offers a course in specialized translation and conference interpreting for the technical, scientific, economic, legal, bio-medical, healthcare and social services sectors. In 2021, SSML Rimini at the Fondazione Unicampus San Pellegrino (FUSP) organized a webinar offering an introduction to medical interpreting (6 hours), but there is no mention of any further webinars of this kind being organized in the following year. The same institute organized two postgraduate Public Service Interpreting (PSI) courses, with on-the-job experiences in the *questura* (police headquarters) in Rimini and the hospitals of Rimini, Ancona and Bologna (academic years 2007–2008, 2008–2009 and 2009–2010).

As well as the courses mentioned above, there are also advanced training courses (*Alta Formazione*), devoted to medical interpreting, as in the case of the SSML in Naples, which offers a course on healthcare cultural mediation, or UNINT in Rome, which is planning to offer an advanced training course on medical interpreting in English, French, German (not yet started). Università degli Studi di Bari Aldo Moro (UNIBA) also offers an advanced training course for ethno-clinical intercultural mediators that exclusively focuses on theoretical aspects of mediation in the socio-healthcare and migration sector (without any dialogue interpreting practice) and is conceived for mediators working in the healthcare sector. UNIBO has recently launched a life-long learning programme on linguistic assistance in the legal and social-healthcare sector (not yet started). Such courses have a duration ranging from 175 hours to 7 months.

Over 100 university programmes (BA and MA) in Italy have been analysed and mapped, including the language combinations offered. Within these programmes, almost all of the courses that include some form of medical interpreting are compulsory, as medical interpreting is almost always taught in dialogue interpreting courses, which themselves are compulsory. The number of ECTS credits awarded for these courses vary, but in general, 10–12 ECTS are awarded to the entire course that includes medical interpreting. The most common language combination taught in Italy is Italian-English, while language combinations involving the main Western European languages (French, German, Spanish, Portuguese) are also very common. Over the last few decades, there has been an increase in programmes offering Russian, Chinese and Arabic, but these are frequently chosen as C languages.[6] The language combination Albanian<>Italian is

---

6   Italian<>Arabic is offered in seventeen interpreting/language mediation courses in fourteen universities; Chinese<>Italian is offered in twenty interpreting/language mediation courses in nineteen universities; Russian<>Italian is offered in twenty-eight interpreting/language mediation courses in twenty-two universities.

being offered on an interpreting/language mediation course at one university; Serbo-Croatian<>Italian is being offered in four interpreting/language mediation courses at four universities; some BA courses (such as Linguistic and Intercultural Mediation at the Università La Sapienza) offer language courses in Ukrainian, Hindi, Greek, Czech, Slovakian and Hungarian, but while written mediation is mentioned, no reference is made to dialogue interpreting or oral mediation courses. Some BA and MA programmes (Modern Languages, European and American Languages and Literatures) also offer languages such as Arabic, Chinese, Korean, Japanese, Hindi and Persian, but, here again, no reference is made to dialogue interpreting or oral mediation courses.

As for the methods and resources used in the teaching of these courses, specific information is hard to find, but in general terms they include memory exercises, terminology exercises, and, most prominently, role plays simulating or reproducing real interactions.

In conclusion, the only university courses currently devoted specifically to medical interpreting are advanced training courses (*Alta Formazione*). Migrants' needs are usually met with training organized by regional bodies, which often lack the adequate focus on language, ethics and specific skills. There is, therefore, a gap that could be filled by offering medical interpreting/mediation courses that could also apply to minority languages, with methods and content being conveyed through a *lingua franca*, enabling the skills and knowledge learned to be transferred to less common languages.

If we compare the needs and expectations for medical interpreting, it seems clear that the university courses offered do not meet the market needs, which are dictated by the flows of tourists and migrants to Italy, a country that attracts a large number of people of different origins. Italy has always been a major tourist destination, attracting millions of tourists each year; according to the Ministry of the Interior and the Italian National Institute of Statistics, in 2019 there were 428.8 million overnight stays by tourists in Italy, almost half of which were by international visitors (Ministero dell'interno 2019, Istat). With 29 million overnight stays, Rome was the main tourist destination, followed by Venice and Milan (both 12.1 million). The largest number of international visitors were from Germany (27.1 per cent), the United States, France, the United Kingdom (ca. 6.5 per cent), the Netherlands, Switzerland, Liechtenstein and Austria (ca. 5 per cent). Rome and other historical cities are not the only tourist destinations in Italy, a country famous for its small historical towns, countryside, and coastal and mountain destinations. Given the number of foreign tourists year-round in major tourist destinations, the health system has a constant need for language support. Furthermore, besides tourism, Italy is also a destination country for migrants from different parts of the world. A first large flow of migrants reached Italy from Eastern Europe after the fall of the Berlin wall and the collapse of the Soviet Union. In particular, large communities from Romania, Poland and Albanian (whose presence in Eastern, Central and Southern Italy has deep roots, with Albanian-speaking communities present since the fifteenth century) settled in Italy in the early 1990s. In recent years, Italy has also become one of the main European destinations for migrants fleeing conflict and poverty in many parts of the world. Migrants mainly reach Italy by sea, landing on the southern shores of Sicily and Calabria. Most of the industrial production is nevertheless located in Northern Italian regions, so once arrived and given permission to stay, a large number of migrants head north. The Italian National Institute of Statistics (Istat) regularly issues reports on the migrant population residing in Italy and the languages spoken. According to Istat, as shown in Table 2.4, Romanian is the largest linguistic community in Italy, followed by Arabic (including all regional varieties), Albanian, Spanish (mostly Latin American varieties), Chinese, Russian, Ukrainian, French, Serbian-Croatian, Polish, English, Bengali, Filipino, Sinhalese and others.

Looking at the information in Table 2.4, apparently, the language combinations offered in interpreting/language mediation courses (both BA and MA) in Italy do not match the language spoken by the largest foreign nationals' communities in Italy who are likely to need language mediation in the healthcare sector. Language combinations offered at university level seem to more closely reflect business needs than social needs. This is probably also linked to the competition among universities, as they try to offer the best and brightest career opportunities to their students. When it comes to interpreting in healthcare settings, the language combinations offered are mainly oriented to cover the needs of tourists,

Table 2.4. Foreign citizens living in Italy (aged 6 or above) according to their first language

Original language	Percentage	Absolute values
Romanian	21.89	798,364
Arabic	13.1	476,721
Albanian	10.5	380,361
Spanish	7.0	255,459
Italian	4.5	162,148
Chinese	4.4	159,597
Russian	3.5	126,849
Ukrainian	3.3	119,883
French	3.2	116,287
Serbian Croatian Bosnian Montenegrin	2.6	93,289
Polish	2.4	87,283
English	2.1	76,693
Bengali	1.5	55,464
Filipino	1.9	70,161
Sinhalese	1.4	49,473
Other language	16.8	611,175
Total	*100.0*	*3,639,227*

Source: Istat (2020)

rather than of migrants. English, French and Spanish are often used as a *lingua franca* in healthcare settings, but migrants are not always proficient in these languages. Migrants' language needs in healthcare institutions are mostly covered by intercultural mediators who are often themselves migrants willing to help members of their own ethnic community or people sharing the same language to have full access to healthcare services. They have often attended courses for intercultural mediators offered at regional level (450–600-hour courses authorized or funded by regional authorities), in which they gain insight into legislation, culture, and in some cases (and to a lesser extent) linguistic skills. These mediators are usually welcomed in healthcare settings because in most cases they cover real language needs. It is worth noting that it is difficult for universities to offer language combinations matching the migrants' needs, because migration flows change over time and from region to region.

3.1.3. Romania

Through our research on university curricula in Romania (as presented on the universities websites in 2022), we identified forty-five programmes (twenty-two BA and twenty-three MA programmes) offering interpreting, specialized translation and/or intercultural communication in twenty-five universities.

No medical interpreting training course is currently offered in Romania and, other than the extracurricular module to be implemented in the wake of the ReACTMe project, there do not seem to be any concrete plans to fill this gap, despite the clear need (see immigration figures below). This is not to say that Romanian students do not have any opportunity to acquire the knowledge and skills they would need when working in healthcare contexts. To obtain a more nuanced overview of the situation and thus highlight both the potential of the Romanian higher education institutions (HEIs) to accommodate more specialized training and the additions to be made to the curricula, the details of current situation need to be examined.

There are currently two MA programmes in conference interpreting, six in translation and interpreting (either conference interpreting or public service interpreting, the distinction is not made) and fifteen in specialized translation, as well as fourteen BA programmes providing interpreter training,[7] all of which offer consecutive interpreting courses and some even simultaneous courses. Dialogue interpreting, on the other hand, is not taught in these programmes, at least not as a separate subject. Specialized translation courses both at BA and MA level are common, sometimes with a dedicated medical module, and ethics in translation and/or interpreting is taught in all the MA programmes. As for the language combinations within the programmes, English and French are offered by all universities; Spanish

---

7   The curricula of two degree programmes were not available online.

and German come second, while Italian is offered by a few programmes at BA level. In addition to these languages, one MA programme offers Russian, and one BA programme offers Turkish. While Romanian is the A language for most programmes, there are also three particular cases: one BA and two MA programmes with Hungarian (explicitly stated as an A language for two programmes; the third does not mention if Hungarian is an A, B or C language). BA degrees in rare languages (Croatian, Serbian) are also offered by one university. Degrees in Arabic, Chinese, Persian, Ukrainian and several other languages are available, notably at the Universitatea din București (UniBuc) and Universitatea Babeș-Bolyai (UBB), but they focus on the respective languages and literatures and provide no specialized translation or interpreting classes, so these were not included in our analysis. However, the existence of such programmes is still relevant for us, in that their graduates could potentially be trained as interpreters for medical settings in a postgraduate course, and thus help to meet the need in this area. The fact that numerous languages are taught in HEIs is, for Romania, an asset that cannot be ignored. As far as linguistic and cultural mediation is concerned, a BA programme does exist in the Academy of Economics in Bucharest, but it focuses on business communication and no course in interpreting is provided.

It must be said that many of the degrees analysed – even at BA level – mention 'interpreter' as one of the professions to which graduates in languages can aspire; from this it can be inferred that universities consider interpreting to be an attractive option for potential candidates, although the curricula are not, in some cases, convincing. As many BA programmes offer consecutive interpreting classes, it is reasonable to assume that graduates have at least an idea about the techniques and the potential difficulties of interpreting. Moreover, most degree programmes offer courses in specialized language, specialized translation (in some cases, medical) and terminology, which could serve as the basis for appropriate terminology management skills and could lead to a certain awareness of the pitfalls of inappropriate equivalences. Nevertheless, few degrees seem to have a realistic approach to teaching interpreting: in some cases, consecutive and simultaneous interpreting are taught in the same semester, and while many BA programmes offer training in simultaneous interpreting, often little time (one or two semesters) is allotted to interpreting practice and this training occurs too early in the programme (in the second year of some BAs), as we could see in the curricula. Furthermore, most of the programmes mix interpreting with translation, thus leaving insufficient time to devote to either of the two skillsets. Only two MA programmes are specifically focused on conference interpreting, those at UniBuc (with one specialized translation course in the curriculum) and at UBB. The Universitatea Tehnică de Construcții din București (UTCB), on the other hand, provides public service translation courses, a subject not available in other Romanian HEIs. Given the wide range of languages studied at UniBuc and UBB at both BA and MA level and in departments other than translation and interpreting departments, it seems that in these three establishments the pedagogical and human potential for developing a medical interpreting module – ideally in collaboration – might be available.

Admission to the degree programmes analysed within this project is open to anyone who fulfils certain academic requirements (e.g. holding a BA degree for MA programmes, and sometimes passing an admission exam to test the level of linguistic and/or general knowledge), but no specific path was identified for people with professional experience and with languages of limited diffusion in their combination who could be trained as interpreters. The only option for such individuals is to fulfil the academic requirements, train with the languages offered within the programmes and then transfer their skills to other language combinations. This is the case for people with other linguistic backgrounds, such as Hungarian, German, Ukrainian, etc., who have a native level of Romanian.

To sum up this document analysis, there appears to be a human and academic potential to provide training in medical interpreting in Romania. An elective module for interpreting and translation students or a continuous professional development module for active interpreters (organized as a hybrid or online course) are likely to be good starting points. Ideally, experienced trainers from the universities with a tradition in training interpreters should collaborate in delivering courses and creating pedagogical resources with Romanian as a working language.

Table 2.5. Interpreting and translation-related degrees at UniBuc, UBB and UTCB

University	Degree	Courses related to interpreting and specialized translation	Languages (C)
Universitatea din București (UniBuc)	BA in Translation and Interpretation	Specialized Languages Interpreting Practice Theory of Communications and Interpreting Practice Theory and Practice of Translation Internship / Translation portfolio, interpreting	English, French, Spanish, German, Italian, Russian
	BA in Applied Modern Languages	Theory of Translation Terminology	English, French, Spanish, German, Italian, Russian Slovak, Polish, Croatian, Czech
	MA in Conference Interpreter Training	Introduction to Consecutive Interpreting Consecutive Interpreting with Notes Internship (Community Interpreting) Terminology and Term Standardization Consecutive Interpreting with Notes Simultaneous Interpreting A Legal Perspectives on the Translation and Interpreting Profession in the European Context	English, French, Spanish, German

Table 2.5. Continued

University	Degree	Courses related to interpreting and specialized translation	Languages (C)
	MA in Specialized Translation and Terminological Studies	Terminology and Term Standardization Translation and Terminology Practice/Specialized Translation Portfolio Specialized Translation (scientific, technical, and media modules)	English, French, Spanish, German, Italian, Russian
	MA in Applied Russian. Translation Techniques	Theory and Practice of Translation Business Communication Specialized Language Workshop Stylistics of Specialized Language Specialized Terminologies Specialized Translation (*sic*) Workshop (Consecutive, Simultaneous)	Russian
Universitatea Babeș-Bolyai (UBB)	BA in Applied Modern Languages	Introduction to Translation Techniques. Written and Oral Communication Translation. Linguistic and Cultural Mediation Specialized Translation Introduction to Consecutive Interpreting Introduction to Terminology Terminology	English, French, Spanish, German, Italian

(continued)

Table 2.5. Continued

University	Degree	Courses related to interpreting and specialized translation	Languages (C)
	MA in Conference Interpreting	Consecutive Interpretation without Notes Interpreting Techniques Consecutive Interpretation with Notes Simultaneous Interpreting Theory of Interpretation Simultaneous with text	English, French, Spanish
	Main Translation Studies and Terminology	Contemporary Theories of Translation Terminology Professional Simulation. Project Management Audio-visual Translation. Subtitling/Localization. Specialized Translation (Legal, Healthcare, Economics, Science and Technology). Translation Project Translation A European Profession	English, French, Spanish
Universitatea Tehnică de Construcţii din Bucureşti (UTCB)	BA: Translation and Interpreting	Terminology Technical Specialized Translation Theory and Practice of Translation Lexicological Structures and Terminology – Engineering (elective) Theory of Communication and Interpreting Techniques Translation Portfolio / Glossaries / Interpreting	English, French, Spanish, German

Table 2.5. Continued

University	Degree	Courses related to interpreting and specialized translation	Languages (C)
	MA: Specialized Translation and Interpreting	Practical Course of Consecutive Interpreting Technical and Scientific Specialized Translation Intercultural Communication Lexicological Structures and Terminology – Engineering Practical Course in Specialized Translation for Public Services Risk Management in Translation Simultaneous Interpreting for International Relations Practical Course in Simultaneous Interpreting	English, French, Spanish, German

Source: Own elaboration based on UniBuc, UBB and UTCB websites

When designing solutions, it is important to take into consideration the reality of the demand, which means that training in less widely taught languages should be ensured. According to the Eurostat (2022: online) report 'Migration and migrant population statistics' updated on 27 April 2022, Romania is mainly a country of emigration,[8] but despite this still receives a significant number of immigrants. On 1 January 2021, 3.6 per cent of the population was foreign-born, of which 10.6 per cent in Italy, 8.8 per cent in Moldova, 7.4 per cent in Turkey, 5.8 per cent in France, 5.2 per cent in China and 62.5 per cent in other states. To this, one should add the increasing number of foreign tourists coming to Romania. According to the National Institute of Statistics, in May 2022, 858,300 foreigners were accommodated in hotels and similar facilities, representing 16.5 per cent of the total number of tourists and a 40.9 per cent increase with respect

---

8   Moreover, according to the same report, 'Romanian, Polish, Italian and Portuguese citizens were the four biggest groups of EU citizens living in other EU Member States on 1 January 2021', which confirms that healthcare interpreters with Romanian in their language combination are needed in various EU countries.

to May 2021. In total, 1,059,200 foreigners entered Romania in May 2022, a 153.3 per cent increase compared to May 2021 (INSSE 2022). No official statistics exist, but the president of FPTR, the Federation of Romanian Employers' Associations, estimates that 20,000 medical tourists come to Romania annually (Federația Patronatelor din Turismul Românesc 2020). In addition, with the war that broke out between Russia and Ukraine on 24 February 2022, and the tens of thousands of Ukrainian refugees crossing the Romanian borders (ReliefWeb 2022), the need for interpreting services (including medical interpreting) with Ukrainian, but also with English and Russian as vehicular languages, increased steeply in a very short period, thus highlighting the existing shortcomings in terms of interpreter training.

3.2. Interpreters' and interpreter trainers' perspectives on medical interpreting training

3.2.1. Focus groups in Spain

Four focus groups were conducted in Spain with a total of twenty-five participants: two with professional medical interpreters (six and seven participants, respectively), one with interpreter trainers (eight participants) and one with heads of translation and interpreting departments or directors of translation and interpreting degree programmes (four participants).

According to the participants in the various focus groups, there are many differences between medical interpreters and interpreters working in other settings, especially due to the medical interpreter's relation with both parties, their physical contact with them and the emotional implications. Additionally, participants felt that, due mainly to the asymmetrical relationship between the parties already mentioned by several authors (Angelelli 2004a; Valero-Garcés 2007; Pilnick and Dingwall 2011; García-Izquierdo and Montalt 2022), a fact that is less frequent in other settings, such as conference interpreting, for example, medical interpreters perform many tasks that other interpreters would not perform, such as creating an initial climate of trust or reassuring patients.

Another difference mentioned by participants was related to the specific requirements of interpreting in healthcare settings. Participants in the focus groups thought that interpreters of all kinds share the basic techniques and competences, but that there are differences, for example, concerning the specialized terminology or the context in which they work and its protocols. Another important differentiating factor mentioned by several trainers and interpreters was the unexpected situations that may arise in healthcare settings, which result in a consequent lack of specific preparation and the need to make decisions at short notice. Finally, the lack of professional recognition of medical interpreters in Spain compared to conference interpreters was highlighted by the interpreters participating in the focus groups.

Unsurprisingly, the differences noted in the focus groups led to a consensus that specific training is required for medical interpreters. Most heads of department and trainers thought that the best option would be to offer specialized training at master's or postgraduate level. Interpreters, on the other hand, believed that this training should not necessarily be provided through a full university degree, but could be a shorter course/module, as authors like Vargas-Urpí (2016) or Burdeus-Domingo et al. (2021) have also recommended. Furthermore, based on their experience in the field, participants suggested that training for healthcare professionals who work with interpreters should also be organized.

Concerning the competences that, in the participants' view, medical interpreters should acquire and develop, the balance between empathy and the ability to deal with the emotional impact of medical interpreting was considered essential if the interpreter is to avoid stress and trauma. According to the participants, thematic and contextual knowledge (healthcare systems, procedures and documents, structure of the consultation, basics of the medical interview, history taking, diagnosis, etc.) are also very important.

Participants from all groups mentioned the importance of linguistic and cultural competence. Concerning linguistic competence, participants believed that knowing the standard variety of the two languages involved would not be enough. This is in line with Angelelli (2019: 91), who states that healthcare providers and patients 'belong to different speech communities'. Therefore, knowing not only the specialized terminology used in healthcare settings but also different registers and varieties, including main dialects, was, in their opinion, crucial. As for culture, participants considered it necessary for interpreters to be aware of the link between cultural patterns, and beliefs and customs related to health.

The ability to interpret using different modes – mainly dialogue, consecutive and sight translation – was also mentioned by almost every participant. Finally, more general competences were also pointed out; these included turn-taking management, the ability to make the parties understand the interpreter's role, the capacity to negotiate and argue and assertiveness.

Regarding the methods and resources for training, online platforms (e.g. Linkterpreting, <http://linkterpreting.uvigo.es>), terminology exercises, role plays, videos with examples of medical interviews, or mock exams provided by some certification bodies of the United States and the United Kingdom seem to be commonly used by the trainers participating in the focus groups. In relation to role plays, according to the trainers, involving healthcare professionals in the simulations (Creeze et al. 2015; Sanz-Moreno 2017; Krystallidou et al. 2018) and practicing with non-scripted role plays would be ideal. Furthermore, in general, participants noted a lack of materials that are linguistically and culturally adapted to the Spanish context, an issue that is expected to (at least partially) have been solved with the materials developed within the ReACTMe project and gathered in its learning platform.

Finally, on the subject of language combinations, the ideas shared by the heads of departments and the trainers were the following:

- English and French are offered in the majority of university-level programmes in translation and interpreting. This could be useful for communication with tourists and some migrants living in coastal zones of Spain or even, if varieties are studied, with migrants from some African countries, but this offer is insufficient;
- the modern standard Arabic taught in university classrooms does not correspond with the Arabic dialects spoken by the immigrant communities living in Spain; the same may also be applied to Chinese;

- the knowledge acquired by interpreting students related to their C and D languages is not usually enough to interpret in healthcare settings.

In short, according to the focus group participants, the language combinations offered do not match the language needs of Spanish public services in general, and of healthcare services in particular.

3.2.2. Focus groups in Italy

Four focus groups were carried out in Italy with twenty-two participants: two with professional medical interpreters (twelve participants in total) and two with interpreter trainers and heads of translation and interpreting departments, or directors of Translation and Interpreting degrees (ten participants in total).

Before getting into the actual results of our research in Italy, a clarification needs to be made about how the professional role which is the subject of this research is denominated. So far, reference has been made to medical interpreters, but in Italy there are also other designations for those working in community settings and facilitating communication between people speaking a different language: linguistic/linguistic-cultural/intercultural/social/sociocultural mediator. Whether this is just a matter of denomination or a more substantial difference has been investigated by scholars (Pöchhacker 2008, 2012; Rudvin and Tomassini 2008; Garzone 2009; Amato 2012; Falbo 2013; Baraldi and Gavioli 2015; Morelli 2017; Niemants 2017) and this distinction also emerged several times in the focus groups held both with trainers and professional interpreters, where a purported difference in the roles was emphasized by some and denied by others. What emerged from the opinions expressed in the focus groups was that some conceived interpreters as mere translators of words, while mediators were seen as professionals more involved with cultural background and knowledge, being able to bridge the communication between doctors and patients. As such, it may be useful to provide here some information to clarify the situation. In the literature, scholars seem to agree on the fact that in the field of translation and interpreting it is necessary to add the dimension of culture to that of language; a number of authors have come to reject a purely linguistic view of translation (and interpreting) as too narrow (Pöchhacker 2008), and therefore, interpreting should already be equated with mediation. The situation in Italy appears to be more complex than that (Dallari et al. 2005; Mack 2005; Pöchhacker 2008; Rudvin and Tomassini 2008). The terms *mediazione linguistica / linguistico-culturale / interculturale / sociale / socioculturale* [linguistic / linguistic-cultural / intercultural / social / sociocultural mediation] were introduced in the 1990s. This may be linked to the university reform introduced in Italy in those years and the need to design interpreting and translation curricula for BA and MA levels; the contents of BA degrees being of a general nature, the BA courses (L12 class of degree programme) were named 'Linguistic Mediation' and offer only an introduction to interpreting (if any), namely dialogue interpreting, whereas simultaneous and consecutive forms of interpreting were left to the MA programmes (LM94 class of degree programmes). Such a difference between the designation of interpreters and mediators may also originate in the mention of intercultural mediators in the legal framework, first in Law no. 40 of 6 March 1998, followed by Legislative Decree 286/98, Italian Presidential Decree 394/99, Legislative Decree no. 13 of 16 January 2013 and others (Albertini 2010; Amato and Garwood 2011; Merlini 2019). Such laws provided for new professional figures to bridge the existing gap in linguistic assistance for migrants. Indeed, in those years, after being a country of emigration for more than a century, Italy was faced with a new phenomenon, that of extensive immigration. Migrants on the Italian territory needed assistance, including on medical issues, to overcome linguistic and cultural barriers, and such services were offered by NGOs or community associations and agencies, ad hoc interpreters and often by migrants themselves with little or no training in the field, but with an extensive knowledge of the migrants' culture of origin, allowing them to bridge communication, whereas universities and scholars continued to focus on conference interpreting. Hence the perceived difference between *interpreting* as an activity merely limited to language often provided by highly educated professionals, and *intercultural mediation*, including also interpreting, often offered by people with little training but with a knowledge of minority languages and cultures operating mainly in the legal or healthcare sector. Interestingly, in 2015, a UNI norm was introduced in Italy in an attempt to determine standards for the translation and interpreting sector (which was and remains without any official regulation), as envisaged by Law 4/2013.[9] The norm was drafted by a working group made up of professional associations, some universities with a long tradition of teaching interpreting and translation, a representative of the European Commission's Directorate-General for Translation (DGT), members of the UNI working groups and a representative of the CNCU (National Council of Consumers and Users). Following a consultation process involving the collection of comments from interested parties, the norm was published, thus offering to users and professionals an impartial and recognized tool for the description of the professional activities of translators and interpreters. The norm describes the set of knowledge, abilities and skills of professional translators and interpreters based on EU recommendations. The norm was also reviewed in 2022, and according to the reviewed text, interlinguistic and intercultural mediation indicates *all* translation and interpreting professional activities and should be conceived as a hypernym of such activities. In the norm, therefore, the definition includes all oral and written forms of communication among people who do not share the same culture and language, thus rejecting *de facto* any distinction between interpreters translating words and mediators translating culture, and offering a new perspective in the ongoing debate.

When, during the focus groups, professionals and trainers were asked if medical interpreters' work differs from other forms of interpreting and if specialized training was necessary, almost all interviewees agreed that medical interpreting differs from other forms of interpreting, such as conference interpreting or interpreting in other dialogic settings (the legal setting, for example). Besides the area-specific terminology, the main differences identified by trainers lie in the stressful and highly emotional situations the interpreters are faced with, the cultural taboos and implications surrounding the body and health, the asymmetry in communication, the need to manage empathy, a personal history/background allowing the

---

9 UNI is a private non-profit Italian association establishing standards for different industries.

interpreters to relate to the situation, the tremendous responsibility of dealing with the health and dignity of another person, the specificity of the setting itself, with its various wards and departments with which the interpreters have to familiarize themselves, soft skills and psychological impacts. As a result of these differences, according to the participants, interpreters working in the healthcare sector should go beyond the linguistic barrier and deploy their cultural knowledge and emotional maturity. Several trainers stressed that the asymmetric communication that medical interpreters have to bridge is a peculiar feature of the hospital setting. However, it was also underlined that once interpreters are trained, they should be able to adjust their skills to the specific working environment, and participants stressed that interpreters and mediators should not be considered as two different and opposite figures (Dallari et al. 2005; Baraldi and Gavioli 2012; Falbo 2013). Professional interpreters mentioned the same features in their focus groups, but dwelt more specifically on the bond of trust that medical interpreters have to create with doctors and patients (Angelelli 2004b; Amato et al. 2018; Wadensjö 2018) (both doctors and patients need to be assured that the interpreter has everything under control, they have to feel comfortable with a third party being present at such a delicate moment, etc.); it was also stressed that a good relationship can affect the outcome of the visit and the diagnosis, and that the relational aspect is what really makes the difference between court/medical interpreting and conference interpreting. For some professional interpreters, it is the settings and not the skills that are different from other forms of dialogic interpreting, because interpreters have to familiarize themselves with the tools, procedures and hierarchies of the different departments, and even with the sounds, smells and emotions experienced in a hospital ward. Some highlighted that working in a hospital means being asked to interpret for a gynaecologist, a cardiologist and a neurologist on the same day, stressing how different the terminology and procedures can be in the different departments. The psychological and emotional burden was also mentioned by almost all professionals, as medical interpreters are not isolated in a booth as in a conference, they are physically sharing the same space with the doctor and the patient and have to work in very delicate situations, especially when working with children and oncological patients, sometimes having to deliver bad news to the patient. Interpreters therefore have to learn how to establish a relationship with the patients without being overwhelmed by their individual situations.

In light of all the specificities mentioned above, trainers and professional interpreters were also invited to discuss and exchange their views and experiences on the need for specialized training, which was acknowledged by all as a necessity. All participants agreed that professional interpreters working in hospital settings should be adequately prepared in advance. For example, both trainers and professional interpreters agree that all those working in the medical sector should be taught (at least basic) anatomy and physiology, together with information about not only the main medical procedures, but also administrative and bureaucratic procedures, since these are things they have to deal with in their daily activities with tourists and migrants. Trainers also discussed at length what kind of training is currently being offered in their universities and what would be advisable for the future, suggesting that while it is possible to give some general ideas about the field in BA programme or in the dialogic interpreting course in the MA programme, it is not possible to offer courses devoted entirely to medical interpreting in the ordinary curricula, because it would be too specific, and there is not enough time to offer courses in every specific field. There was a consensus among trainers and professional interpreters that such a course should be offered as an advanced training course to graduate students and to professionals who are already working as interpreters and wish to specialize in the medical field. In this way, it would be possible to focus on all relevant elements for the specific profession. Professionals, in particular, underlined that besides education, internships should also be promoted, because while knowledge of terminology, anatomy and physiology, as well as diagnostic methods and medical procedures is necessary, medical interpreters should also challenge themselves with the hospital settings and its specificities, meaning also tolerating the sight of blood, vomit, people suffering, etc. According to some interpreters and trainers in the focus groups, an advanced training course in medical interpreting could also involve mediators and give them more thorough training on linguistic skills, ethical guidelines, medical notions, etc., thus helping to fill the existing gap.

Both professionals and trainers highlighted the importance of acquiring skills such as stress management, emotional awareness, situational awareness, the ability to adapt and react to individual situations and patients, etc. Something that was stressed by professional interpreters in particular was that students should be prepared to work in emergency situations, which can sometimes require renouncing precision, confidentiality and other prerogatives an interpreter would usually hold for the sake of speed and communication efficiency. Interestingly, some trainers stressed the need for doctors and healthcare staff to be trained in working with interpreters, which is in line with previous research, such as Verrept (2008), to ensure effective communication in mediated interactions. Some successful examples of this nature in the regions of Emilia-Romagna and Liguria were mentioned.

As for methods and resources that can be used in medical interpreting courses, trainers agreed that the most relevant resource is role plays, as was also supported by Valero-Garcés 2008 and Niemants and Bernardi 2021. They also mentioned exercises on the sight translation of documents that are common in the daily activities of interpreters, such as informed consent forms or anamnestic questionnaires used during real interactions, as well as general texts dealing with medicine and health, which can also be useful to master terminology and medical knowledge. In roleplay activities for future medical interpreters, doctor-patient interactions are simulated, with three people acting as doctor, patient and interpreter. Role plays generally simulate routine consultations and also more unexpected situations (e.g. situations that might occur in the emergency department). The importance of preparing students for the asymmetry of communication in the medical field was also stressed, and a new course introduced at the University of Bologna in Forlì was mentioned, where thirty hours on the theory of dialogue interpreting are followed by twenty hours of practice through roleplay exercises in five different languages. Preparatory exercises on medical terminology were also mentioned as an effective learning method.

According to trainers, the resources used often depend on the trainers' experience and field of expertise, and may range from guidelines and specialized texts to transcriptions of authentic (interpreter-mediated) interactions, glossaries, etc. In order to make the most of role plays, trainers also suggested asking students to study the specific condition/symptoms/pathology of the roleplay in advance and to prepare a bilingual glossary with relevant terminology or a list of the most frequent questions asked in such a situation. Playing video recordings of medical consultations in a foreign language (not necessarily interpreter-mediated) was also suggested, so that students can be guided to focus on the general characteristics of such consultations, or video-recorded interpreter-mediated interactions in a different foreign language than that of the course so that they can focus on posture, non-verbal communication, etc. While confirming the prominent use of scripted roleplays as a training method, trainers also underlined the importance of leaving the roleplay open to changes dictated by students' renditions. Trainers also stated that, whenever possible, non-scripted role plays involving real healthcare professionals should also be used, because they are found to be much more stimulating for students and closer to healthcare professionals' real working lives. The need to also train healthcare professionals was once again raised; while successful examples of this were mentioned, they remain only isolated pilot initiatives, locally appreciated by attendees, but lacking coordination and continuity. Finally, it was stressed that training courses on interpreter-mediated intercultural communication could target not only interpreters/mediators, but also medical students.

As it seems, there is a general lack of consistency in training methods and resources used in universities in Italy, as much of this depends on the individual trainers. Some trainers proposed the introduction of telephone interpreting and other forms of remote interpreting in possible interpreting courses, as such forms are becoming increasingly common, especially after the COVID-19 pandemic, and can represent a valid solution for the future, but require different strategies and competences.

3.2.3. Focus groups in Romania

Four focus groups were conducted in Romania with a total of nineteen participants: four with professional medical interpreters (twelve participants in total), and two with higher education policy/decision makers and translation and interpreting trainers (seven participants in total).

The questions asked to the two categories of participants concerned to a large extent similar aspects, but from different perspectives, as can be seen in the Methodology section – with professional interpreters emphasizing the experiences they had and what they had known before and trainers/university representatives concentrating on what can be done from now on – hence the two types of focus groups are presented separately.

Given the demand for medical interpreters, professional interpreters in Romania occasionally work in healthcare settings despite the lack of specific training. Thus, taking the pulse of their experiences was an essential part of our research 'in the field'. Four focus groups were organized and twelve interpreters joined. They shared interesting insights, and unambiguously supported the idea of specialized training in the field.

The existence of differences between medical interpreters and other categories of interpreter was unanimously acknowledged by participants and the list of differences was widely agreed upon: terminology (especially because there are so many specialities), emotional impact, the need to remain in control in tense situations, the difficulties of dealing with dialects and poorly spoken *lingua franca*, a relatively hectic working schedule and the need to always be available. According to participants, specialized training is needed – even for those who are already professional interpreters – on the preparation of terminology and on the ethical issues specific to the field. Participants felt that a one-year MA programme would be suitable, but that a (possibly elective) course for conference interpreting students would also be a viable option. Whatever the form selected, participants believed in the importance of collaboration with healthcare professionals to make the training more relevant.

When asked about the competences required of a medical interpreter, participants mentioned precision, mastery of terminology, good linguistic skills in general, appropriate personality, background knowledge, good stress management, coping strategies, and flexibility. Most importantly, they highlighted the need for an authoritative body that would be in charge of assessing and acknowledging these competences.

In the meantime, as our research within the ReACTMe project showed (see Chapter 1, Section 4 in this volume), ad hoc medical interpreters are frequently used in Romanian healthcare services. Based on their own experiences, the professional interpreters participating in the focus groups said that this could be due to a range of different reasons of varying complexity:

- lack of information: people usually do not know that this work should be carried out by a trained professional, or they do not know how to find an interpreter;
- patients often speak basic English and are not aware of the limits of their knowledge;
- financial aspects: legislation concerning interpreters is scarce, the fees offered ridiculously low, and some patients might not be able to afford the interpreting fees normally requested on the interpreting market;
- sometimes medical professionals speak the patient's mother tongue (in the case of healthcare professionals belonging to Romania's ethnic minorities or of those who came from abroad to study in the country and then decided to stay after graduation);
- in the case of asylum seekers, it is often a peer who provides interpretation.

The issue of ethical guidelines is sensitive and the Romanian interpreters working in healthcare settings are in the difficult position of not having one set of officially acknowledged guidelines. Only patchy solutions are found, and not always. Some NGOs have ethical codes that interpreters can use; to give one example, CNRR, the Romanian National Council for Refugees, used to organize an annual seminar in which ethical issues were also discussed. One interpreter who worked in the UK followed a British code, while another, working with Arabic, said she uses her cultural knowledge to prevent possible ethical issues. Based on real-life examples, all the interpreters said that most often one needs to adapt and to use common sense and one's knowledge of interpreting to deal with delicate situations or ethical dilemmas.

As for the role of the interpreter, participants stated that it is not always understood. It became clear from the discussion that an understanding of the role really depends on individual doctors and patients. The interviewees shared experiences of doctors who thought they understood patients without speaking their language, or who did not ask for an interpreter on time. Briefing and debriefing are not common practices.

The Romanian team also organized two focus groups with higher education policy/decision makers and translation and interpreting trainers (attended by a total of seven participants). The participants of these focus groups confirmed the data from the analysis of their universities' curricula, including language combinations, and added useful information indicating an interest in the medical field: at UTCB, trainers are free to select the fields on which they focus within the course on translation for public services; at UBB, students benefited from two short healthcare modules delivered by a trainer from Universidad San Jorge (USJ), in 2015 and 2018 respectively (for an analysis of the impact of the second module, see Nevado Llopis and Pelea 2019), while second-year students in conference interpreting have two themed weeks on medical interpreting, and interpreter trainers have useful contacts with Romanian graduates of Philology faculties, who do not have formal training in the field, but have rich experience as healthcare interpreters in the UK.

Participants considered the main differences between conference/business/legal interpreters and medical interpreters to be terminology and emotional involvement, with one experienced trainer and head of an MA programme stressing that there are also similarities between the legal context – which is more often covered in interpreter training – and healthcare. Participants unanimously agreed on the need for medical interpreters to have specialized training. The discussion on the most appropriate training led to the conclusion that the MA and postgraduate levels are the most likely to yield results, but that a full MA programme might be too much. One interesting question arose that still needs to be answered: would it be enough to have one MA providing medical interpreting training for the entire country? A realistic suggestion was for the Centre for Language Industries at UBB to organize an advanced training course or summer course to which trainers from other universities could also contribute, then to build on this experience to ensure regular instruction.

As for the pedagogical aspects, participants listed several competences that a medical interpreter needs to acquire: good communication skills, mastery of working languages, minimal training in healthcare/basic medical knowledge (especially anatomy), rich background knowledge (even more important than for conference interpreting, according to one participant), and all the skills usually required in public service interpreting. In this context, it was stressed that training should emphasize the idea that the interpreter needs to stay 'in the shadows', to be simply an interface, as well as the importance of confidentiality. Participants agreed that the main training methods used were role plays, terminological exercises and glossaries, while the presence of medical professionals during training activities was considered essential.

The focus groups with professional interpreters, interpreter trainers and representatives of HEIs were an opportunity to find out even more information than we had initially anticipated and to collect precious suggestions for implementing a medical interpreting module in Romania. It is useful to note that two public hospitals in Cluj-Napoca already have contracts with an interpreter (who had a job interview before being accepted), and thus doctors can contact her when they need interpreting services with her language combination, and also that medical tourism is, at least in Cluj-Napoca, creating further demand. Several concrete suggestions were made during these focus groups with respect to the training of medical interpreters and the establishment of organized interpreting services (as also explained in Chapter 3, Section 6 in this volume).

The last question addressed to trainers and HEI representatives was whether the language combinations currently offered in interpreter training by Romanian universities answer the linguistic and cultural needs in the Romanian healthcare services and the answer was that they clearly do not, as can also be inferred by the recent demographic statistics quoted above.

4. Conclusions

This second year of our project provided essential information for a deeper understanding of both the strengths and weaknesses of the current situation in terms of the training for and practice of interpreting in healthcare settings in the three participating countries. Having identified both the potential and the needs, it is possible to design the next steps to be taken individually, in each country, and together, starting from the cooperation already in place through the ReACTMe consortium, to capitalize on the complementary experiences and linguistic demands.

Our results indicate a series of similarities between the three countries, as well as differences that could, in certain respects, serve as models to follow in the future.

The need for medical interpreting and the fact that this need is currently insufficiently fulfilled were acknowledged throughout all focus groups. Two main categories of beneficiaries are concerned, to different extents: tourists and migrants, the latter having a much more diverse linguistic profile and being less likely to speak a *lingua franca*. Universities, however, only partially respond to this situation. In Spain, there are very few university courses focusing only on medical interpreting. Interpreting in healthcare settings is frequently studied in courses with a broader scope (public service interpreting, intercultural mediation, or even simply interpreting) and most of the time this depends on the individual trainer's choice. Italy is also lacking in university courses devoted specifically to medical interpreting, which is taught only occasionally as part of dialogue interpreting courses and only upon the initiative of individual trainers. In Romania, few programmes allot interpreting the time and attention required for specialized training and none provide specific training for healthcare settings.

Moreover, the languages for which training *is* provided are a long way from covering the actual needs. So, when designing new medical interpreting courses, more attention should be paid to the languages spoken by allophone patients. A potential solution could be to offer courses addressed to a multilingual group of students, with certain activities carried out in small groups distributed by language. Such a course could be provided in a pivot language and contents could easily be transferred to other languages. The course could be offered to graduates of interpreting programmes or professional interpreters wishing to specialize in medicine, and the course content could include medical knowledge and practical sessions with role plays, scripted and non-scripted, and real interpreter-mediated interactions, while the involvement of healthcare professionals in the interpreters' training would be strongly advised. At the same time, courses on how to work with interpreters could also be offered to students of medicine, nursing or other health sciences to raise their awareness on the specificities of interpreter-mediated interactions. A collaboration between trainers with experience in teaching conference or public service interpreting, teachers of languages for medical purposes and healthcare professionals is essential for the success of any such course. The ReACTMe learning platform has provided resources and templates for developing courses of this kind, which hopefully will be implemented in universities, especially since they would fill a significant gap. The training resources on ReACTMe are precious in our contexts, since they are a reliable, open-access training resource for trainers, students and professional interpreters. Additionally, they are particularly adapted to the Spanish variety spoken in Spain (rather than the varieties spoken in the Americas) and the Spanish context; and, in the case of Romania, they are a first, a necessary initial model for creating the resources needed for a fully-fledged course.

Currently, medical interpreting services are only partially provided by professional interpreters: in the healthcare services of some Spanish autonomous communities (Foulquié Rubio et al. 2018), by mediators with training provided by regional courses in Italy and by conference interpreters in Romania. In all three countries, ad hoc solutions are commonplace: relatives, friends, 'bilingual' medical professionals turned interpreters despite the lack of training, machine translation, etc. As became clear in our focus groups, awareness-raising is as urgent as training.

Another aspect that became clear during this year of research is that the three countries studied in the project have complementary profiles and would all gain from cooperating in terms of training. Each country's language is needed in the field of medical interpreting in the other two participating countries, and in most cases the offer does not match the demand (especially for Romanian, as well as Italian – and to a certain extent, Spanish – in Romania). With the remote training experience acquired during the pandemic, it can safely be assumed that a joint programme with trainers and trainees from the three countries is feasible. The Joint Blended Extracurricular Module on Medical Interpreting and the Key elements to be considered when designing a course for medical interpreters (see Chapters 5 and 6) provide an excellent starting point for such cooperation. The advantages are twofold: not only would the trainer pool be richer, but, with the growing role of remote interpreting, trained interpreters in one country could work for clients in the other two using the available technology.

Bibliography

Albertini, Valentina, and Giulia Capitani. 2010. 'La mediazione linguistico-culturale: Stato dell'arte e potenzialità', *I Quaderni del CESVOT* 47. <www.cesvot.it/documentazione/la-mediazione-linguistico-culturale>.

Álvaro Aranda, Cristina, and Raquel Lázaro Gutiérrez. 2021. 'La formación en interpretación sanitaria y su camino hacia la profesionalización: un análisis de itinerarios formativos propuestos desde distintas entidades de España', *Panace@* 22(53), 69–71. <www.tremedica.org/wp-content/uploads/panacea21-53_10_Tribuna_04_AlvaroAranda_LazaroGutierrez.pdf>.

Amato, Amalia. 2012. *L'interprete nel contesto medico*. Bologna: CLUEB.

Amato, Amalia, and Chris Garwood. 2011. 'Cultural mediators in Italy: A new breed of linguists', *InTRAlinea* 16. <www.intralinea.org/archive/article/Cultural_mediators_in_Italy_a_new_breed_of_linguists>.

Amato, Amalia, Michela Bertozzi, Sabine Braun, Gabriel Cabrera Méndez, Enrico Capiozzo, Lisa Danese, Elena Davitti, María Jesús González Rodríguez, Emilia Iglesias Fernández, Juana Muñoz López, Mariachiara Russo, and Nicoletta Spinolo. 2018. *Handbook of Remote Interpreting – SHIFT in Orality*. AMSActa. <www.researchgate.net/publication/335489850_Handbook_of_Remote_Interpreting_-_SHIFT_in_Orality_Erasmus_project>.

Angelelli, Claudia V. 2004a. *Medical Interpreting and Cross-cultural Communication*. New York: Cambridge University Press.

Angelelli, Claudia V. 2004b. *Revisiting the Interpreter's Role: A Study of Conference, Court, and Medical Interpreters in Canada, Mexico, and the United States*. Amsterdam: John Benjamins.

Angelelli, Claudia V. 2019. *Healthcare Interpreting Explained*. New York: Routledge.

ARACIS, Agenția Română de Asigurare a Calității în Învățământul Superior. <www.aracis.ro>.

Baraldi, Claudio, and Laura Gavioli. 2012. 'Understanding coordination in interpreted-mediated interaction', in Claudio Baraldi and Laura Gavioli (eds), *Coordinating Participation in Dialogue Interpreting*. Amsterdam: John Benjamins, 1–22.

Baraldi, Claudio, and Laura Gavioli. 2015. 'Mediation', in F. Pöchhacker (ed.), *The Routledge Encyclopedia of Interpreting Studies*. London: Routledge, 248.

Burdeus-Domingo, Noelia, Suzanne Gagnon, Sophie Pointurier, and Yvan Leanza. 2021. 'Bridges and barriers in public service interpreting training: Instructing non-professional long serving interpreters', *FITISPos International Journal: Public Service Interpreting and Translation* 8, 28–42. <https://doi.org/10.37536/FITISPos-IJ.2021.8.1.267>.

Camacho Sánchez, Fátima. 2019. 'Formación en traducción e interpretación en los servicios públicos en los programas oficiales de grado impartidos en España', *FITISPos International Journal : Public Service Interpreting and Translation* 6, 235–245. <https://ebuah.uah.es/dspace/bitstream/handle/10017/40529/formacion_camacho_FITISPos_2019_6.pdf?sequence=1&isAllowed=y>.

Creeze, Ineke H. M., Holly Mikkelson, and Laura Monzon-Storey. 2015. *Introduction to Healthcare for Spanish-speaking Interpreters and Translators*. Amsterdam: John Benjamins.

Dallari, Giovanna, Debora Previti, and Stefania Ricci. 2005. 'Interprete o mediatore culturale? Le aspettative di un servizio sanitario italiano', in Mariachiara Russo and Gabriele Mack (eds), *Interpretazione di trattativa*. Milan: Hoepli, 183–193.

Eurostat. 2022. 'Migration and migrant population statistics'. <https://ec.europa.eu/eurostat/statistics-explained/index.php?title=Migration_and_migrant_population_statistics#Migration_flows:_Immigrati>.

Falbo, Caterina. 2013. 'Interprete et mediatore linguistico-culturale: Deux figures professionnelles opposées?', in Giovanni Agresti and Cristina Schiavone (eds), *Plurilinguisme et monde du travail: Professions, opérateurs et acteurs de la diversité linguistique*. Rome: Aracne, 253–267.

Federația Patronatelor din Turismul Românesc, 'Străinii cheltuiesc peste 60 de milioane de euro anual pentru intervenții medicale în România'. 2020. <www.fptr.ro/presa/comunicate-de-presa-fptr/strainii-cheltuiesc-peste-60-de-milioane-de-euro-anual-pentru-interventii-medicale-in-romania.aspx>.

Foulquié Rubio, Ana Isabel, Mireia Vargas-Urpí, and María Magdalena Fernández Pérez (eds). 2018. *Panorama de la traducción y la interpretación en los servicios públicos españoles: Una década de cambios, retos y oportunidades*. Granada: Comares.

Fundación Universia. 2022. *Estudios universitarios*. <www.universia.net/es/estudios>.

García-Izquierdo, Isabel, and Vicent Montalt. 2022. 'Cultural competence and the role of the patient's mother tongue: An exploratory study of health professionals' perceptions', *Societies* 12(2), 53. <https://doi.org/10.3390/soci 2020053>.

Garzone, Giuliana. 2009. 'L'interprete e il mediatore: aspetti deontologici', in Donna Miller and Ana Pano (eds), *La geografia della mediazione linguistico-culturale*. Bologna: Alma-DL, 97–116.

Guvernul României. 2022. 'Hotărârea nr. 385/2021 privind domeniile și programele de studii universitare de master acreditate și numărul maxim de studenți ce pot fi școlarizați în anul universitar 2021–2022', Aracis. <www.aracis.ro/wp-cont ent/uploads/2021/04/HG-385-2021-Masterat.pdf>.

Guvernul României. 2022b. 'Hotărârea nr. 883/2021 pentru modificarea anexelor nr. 1–6 la Hotărârea Guvernului nr. 403/2021 privind aprobarea Nomenclatorului domeniilor și al specializărilor/programelor de studii universitare și a structurii instituțiilor de învățământ superior pentru anul universitar 2021–2022', Aracis. <www.aracis.ro/wp-content/uploads/2021/09/883-Hotarare-si-anexe.pdf>.

Guvernul României. 2022c. 'Hotărârea nr. 906/2021 pentru modificarea anexelor nr. 1 și 2 la Hotărârea Guvernului nr. 385/2021 privind domeniile și programele de studii universitare de master acreditate și numărul maxim de studenți ce pot fi școlarizați în anul universitar 2021–2022', Aracis. <www.aracis.ro/wp-content/ uploads/2021/09/906-Hotarare-si-anexe.pdf>.

INE. 2022a. 'Cifras de población (CP) a 1 de enero de 2022. Estadística de migraciones (EM). Año 2021', Instituto Nacional de Estadística. <www.ine.es/ prensa/cp_e2022_p.pdf>.

INE. 2022b. 'Número de turistas según país de residencia', Instituto Nacional de Estadística. <www.ine.es/jaxiT3/Datos.htm?t=10822>.

INSSE. 2022. 'Turismul în luna mai 2022', Institutul Național de Statistică. <https:// insse.ro/cms/sites/default/files/com_presa/com_pdf/turismo5r22_1.pdf>.

Krystallidou, Demi, Myriam Deveugele, Céline Van De Walle, and Evangelia Dougali. 2018. 'Training doctor-minded interpreters and interpreter-minded doctors: First insights into the benefits of collaborative practice in interpreter training', *Interpreting: An International Journal of Research and Practice in Interpreting* 20(1), 126–144. <https://doi.org/10.1075/intp.00005.kry>.

Libera Università di Lingue e Comunicazione IULM, <www.iulm.it/it/myiulm/ corsi/triennali/interpretariato-comunicazione>.

Mack, Gabriele. 2005. 'Interpretazione e mediazione: alcuni riflessioni terminologiche', in Mariachiara Russo and Gabriele Mack (eds), *Interpretazione di trattativa*. Milan: Hoepli, 3–17.

Martin, Anne. 2015. 'La formación en interpretación en España: pasado y presente', *MonTI. Monografías de Traducción e Interpretación* 2, 87–110. <http://dx.doi.org/10.6035/MonTI.2015.ne2.3>.

MECD. 2022. *QUEDU: Qué estudiar y dónde en España*. Ministerio de Educación, Cultura y Deporte. <http://siiu.universidades.gob.es/QEDU/>.

Merlini, Raffaela. 2019. 'Through the looking-glass: Reflections of/on empathy in healthcare', *Cultus* 12, 220–245. <www.cultusjournal.com/files/Archives/Cultus_2019_12_012_Merlini.pdf>.

MIUR. 2022. *Universitaly*. Ministero dell'Università e della Ricerca. <https://www.universitaly.it/>.

Morelli, Mara. 2017. 'Interpreting and mediation: Raising awareness by training', in Letizia Cirillo and Natacha Niemants (eds), *Teaching Dialogue Interpreting*. Amsterdam: John Benjamins, 83–100.

Ministero dell'interno. 2019. *Dossier Viminale*. <www.interno.gov.it/sites/default/files/dossier_viminale_15_agosto_2019.pdf>.

Nevado Llopis, Almudena, and Alina Pelea. 2019. 'Public service interpreting for conference interpreting students: Evaluation of a training module', *The Interpreter's Newsletter* 24, 19–34. <www.openstarts.units.it/bitstream/10077/29522/3/3_Interpreters24_2019.pdf>.

Nevado Llopis, Almudena, and Ana Isabel Foulquié Rubio. 2023. 'Healthcare interpreting training: Present and future at Spanish universities', in Raquel Lázaro Gutiérrez and Cristina Álvaro Aranda (eds), *New Trends in Healthcare Interpreting Studies: An Updated Review of Research in the Field*. Berlin: Springer.

Niemants, Natacha, and Eleonora Bernardi. 2021. 'Interpretare per i servizi socio-sanitari', in Mariachiara Russo (ed.), *Interpretare da e verso l'italiano*. Bologna: Bononia University Press, 395–414.

Niemants, Natacha, and Elizabeth Stokoe. 2017. 'Using the conversational analytical role play method in healthcare interpreter education', in Letizia Cirillo and Natacha Niemants (eds), *Teaching Dialogue Interpreting*. Amsterdam: John Benjamins, 293–322.

Pilnick, Alison, and Robert Dingwall. 2011. 'On the remarkable persistence of asymmetry in doctor/patient interaction: A critical review', *Social Science & Medicine* 72(8), 1374–1382.

Pöchhacker, Franz. 2008. 'Interpreting as mediation', in Carmen Valero-Garcés and Anne Martin (eds), *Crossing Borders in Community Interpreting*. Amsterdam: John Benjamins, 9–26.

Pöchhacker, Franz. 2012. 'Interpreting participation: Conceptual analysis and illustration of the interpreter's role in interaction', in Claudio Baraldi and Laura Gavioli (eds), *Coordinating Participation in Dialogue Interpreting*. Amsterdam: John Benjamins, 45–69.

Relief Web. 2022. *UNHCR Romania: Ukraine Refugee Situation Update, Update #9, 19 August 2022.* <https://reliefweb.int/report/romania/unhcr-romania-ukraine-refugee-situation-update-update-9-19-august-2022>.

Rudvin, Mette, and Elena Tomassini. 2008. 'Migration, ideology and the interpreter-mediator', in Carmen Valero-Garcés and Anne Martin (eds), *Crossing Borders in Community Interpreting.* Amsterdam: John Benjamins, 245–266.

Sanz-Moreno, Raquel. 2017. 'La inclusión del médico en la formación del intérprete en el ámbito sanitario', *Revista Digital de Investigación en Docencia Universitaria* 11(2), 203–222. <http://www.scielo.org.pe/pdf/ridu/v11n2/a13v11n2.pdf>.

SGTMU. 2021. *Datos y cifras del Sistema Universitario Español: Publicación 2020–2021.* Secretaría General Técnica del Ministerio de Universidades. <https://www.universidades.gob.es/wp-content/uploads/2022/11/Datos_y_Cifras_2021_22.pdf>.

Valero-Garcés, Carmen. 2007. 'Doctor–patient consultations in dyadic and triadic exchanges', in Franz Pöchhacker and Miriam Shlesinger (eds), *Healthcare Interpreting: Discourse and Interaction.* Amsterdam: John Benjamins, 165–185.

Valero-Garcés, Carmen. 2008. 'Hospital interpreting practice in the classroom and in the workplace', in Carmen Valero-Garcés and Anne Martin (eds), *Crossing Borders in Community Interpreting.* Amsterdam: John Benjamins, 35–51.

Vargas-Urpí, Mireia. 2016. 'La difícil tarea de dar respuesta a las necesidades de formación en interpretación en los servicios públicos (ISP) en Cataluña: 10 años de avances y retrocesos', *FITISPos International Journal: Public Service Interpreting and Translation* 3, 92–103. <http://hdl.handle.net/10230/28259>.

Verrept, Hans. 2008. 'Intercultural mediation', in Carmen Valero-Garcés and Anne Martin (eds), *Crossing Borders in Community Interpreting.* Amsterdam: John Benjamins, 187–201.

Wadensjö, Cecilia. 2018. 'Involvement, trust and topic control in interpreter-mediated healthcare encounters', *Communication & Medicine* 15(2), 165–176.

ANA ISABEL FOULQUIÉ RUBIO, DONATELLA CIFOLA AND
VERONICA MANOLE

3 Suggestions for the Professionalization of Medical Interpreting in Spain, Italy and Romania

1. Introduction

The ReACTMe project aimed to contribute to the professionalization of medical interpreting in the three countries involved in the project and beyond. More than twenty years ago, Mikkelson (1999: 119) already indicated that the development of public service interpreting as a profession followed the typical pattern of any profession in its infancy, pointing to characteristics such as a 'lack of standards for training and practice' and 'poor working conditions'. Mikkelson (ibid.) also highlighted the importance of the role played by professional associations as well as the need for practitioners to be united and work in the same direction. In the three countries involved in the ReACTMe project, much still needs to be done, as is clear from the previous chapters. There is a lack of standards as regards training and practice, for example, given that there are no specific university courses devoted to the training of medical interpreters. As a result, medical interpreters usually have to learn 'on the job'. This lack of standards is usually linked to the lack of recognition by users and healthcare professionals, who tend to think that this is something that can be done by anyone who speaks two languages. As we have seen in Chapter 1, this is highlighted by healthcare professionals' use of ad hoc interpreters when they need to communicate with allophone patients. This lack of recognition is linked to poor working conditions, including low salaries, isolation from other professionals and difficulties in specializing in just one field.

One of the obstacles to professionalization is the frequent use by healthcare professionals of volunteers or ad hoc interpreters (usually patients' family members, children or friends, or bilingual staff) to communicate with patients. This has somehow 'fulfilled' the need, meaning that some healthcare professionals may not be aware of the important role that professional interpreters play and how they can contribute to effective communication and, consequently, better quality of service.

Based on the information gathered during the three years of the ReACTMe project, this chapter intends to propose ideas for the professionalization of medical interpreting. The information in this chapter is country specific, as there are significant differences among the three countries, especially regarding training. Nevertheless, most of the suggestions for each of the countries could be applied to the other two countries in the project and beyond.

2. Methodology

Four main domains will be taken into account as part of a more comprehensive strategy for professionalization: *training*, *recognition* of the profession, the role of *professional associations*, and the importance of professional standards regarding *working conditions* (payment, working time, preparation, etc.). It is our hope that the further professionalization of medical interpreters will raise awareness among stakeholders (medical staff, administrators, policymakers and patients themselves) of the crucial role played by professional interpreters in healthcare contexts and thus result in a greatly reduced use of ad hoc interpreters or a *lingua franca* to communicate with allophone patients.

Several shortcomings regarding training have already been identified in Chapter 2: the lack of specific training courses in higher education institutions (HEIs), with medical interpreting being studied in all three countries either as part of programmes with a broader scope, such as community or dialogue interpreting, or not studied at all. Our aim, therefore, is to offer suggestions that could be implemented in HEIs in Spain, Italy and Romania, taking into account the feasibility of traditional full university courses and the organization of alternative training opportunities, developed as life-long learning programmes. This aspect will be discussed in Section 3, whereas Section 4 addresses recognition, certification and/or accreditation as a component of the professionalization of medical interpreters. For this set of suggestions, current methods of certification and/or accreditation of interpreters in all three countries will be briefly discussed and more specific types of certifications and/or accreditation will be proposed for medical interpreters. Section 5 is dedicated to the importance of existing associations of professional interpreters, which will be taken into account as crucial actors in the process of professional recognition. In the second half of the twentieth century in particular, powerful associations have played a major role in the professionalization of interpreting, with the International Association of Conference Interpreters (AIIC, <https://aiic.org>) probably the most well-known example. Section 6 provides an overview of active professional associations in all three countries and suggests strategies for their involvement in the professionalization of medical interpreting (through awareness campaigns, workshops, collaboration with medical associations, etc.). Finally, Section 6 will examine the working conditions of both in-house and freelance medical interpreters and the need for standardization. Given the challenging nature of medical interpreting (ethical issues and the emotional load are among the first issues that come to mind), several aspects of the professional routine will be addressed: employment contracts (for permanent staff) or invoicing systems (for freelance interpreters), working time, preparation, debriefing, etc. We will describe the most common methods used by freelance interpreters in the three countries to manage their finances and see whether the same systems can be adopted by medical interpreters. In the case of permanent staff, the ethical nature of the relations between interpreters and their employers (medical staff, hospital administrators, NGOs, etc.) will be addressed. Suggestions for improvement will be made later on in this chapter.

3. Training

When learning how to work in a particular profession, people usually first receive training regarding how that job should be done, and then they start working. In the case of medical interpreting, it has typically been the other way around. People, usually friends or relatives of a given patient, who happen to know a different language from the country's official language, act as interpreters on a voluntary basis and may sometimes then receive some form of training. They do not get paid and, therefore, the work they do is not recognized. This is how medical interpreting started in most countries, such as the United States (Downing and Rushke 2012). In this section we will look at the need for training of medical interpreters, taking as a reference the results obtained during the ReACTMe project in each country.

In most countries, there are no official qualifications to become a professional medical interpreter, and this is also the case in Spain (Pena-Díaz 2018). Spanish universities do, however, offer many bachelor's (BA) degrees in translation and interpreting (see Chapter 2), though very few of these include public service interpreting as a compulsory subject. This type of interpreting is usually included in master's (MA) degrees, but, once more, it is usually an optional subject. In Spain, there is only one BA programme in which public service interpreting is compulsory for all students and only one MA programme specialized in public service interpreting. Moreover, the languages taught at university level do not usually correspond to the demand in healthcare settings. Most universities teach English and French, and while other languages are taught in the BAs or MAs in translation and interpreting, since they are C languages, they are usually not addressed when designing interpreting courses, because students usually get training to interpret into or from their B language. Most languages of lesser diffusion are not included in university curricula, as stated in Chapter 2, and language combinations offered by universities usually meet the needs of tourism and business, while those needed in the healthcare context, such as Romanian or Arabic, are not usually included in the curricula for BA or MA programmes in translation and interpreting.

Given this situation, it is fair to say that many professional interpreters working as medical interpreters have usually received some kind of training in translation and/or interpreting, which provides them with the basic skills needed for interpreting, but have not had training specific to medical interpreting. In the few cases where there are courses related to medical interpreting, it would be a very good idea to include internships in hospitals (similar to those for healthcare students). This would enable interpreting students to learn first-hand about the real challenges of interpreting in medical settings. At the same time, it would raise awareness among healthcare professionals of the need to work with professional interpreters.

3.1. Spain

In Spain, there should be more initiatives including languages of lesser diffusion once the needs of the immigrant population have been analysed. Such initiatives could be promoted by healthcare management areas through non-formal training to adapt them to the situation of each hospital or community, as needs can differ greatly from one place to another. These training initiatives could take the form of short professional courses to provide language of lesser diffusion interpreters with the necessary means to perform the interpreting tasks.

One of the deliverables of the ReACTMe project is the design of a joint blended extracurricular module in medical interpreting. In the case of Spain, Universidad San Jorge (USJ) and Universidad de Murcia (UM) are working together towards the implementation of this module in the two universities. The module designed by the ReACTMe team, which is included in Chapter 6, will be the basis for the development of the training in each country. In the case of Spain, the common language will be Spanish, usually combined with English as the second language (as it is commonly used as a *lingua franca*) and, where possible, other languages, such as Romanian and Arabic (corresponding to the languages spoken by the larger migrant communities) will also be covered, depending on the profiles of participants. As for the content, this extracurricular module will cover a range of topics, including interpreting skills, terminology, ethics and the emotional impact on interpreters, as a result of the different focus groups organized in year 2 of the ReACTMe project. The target group for this training is not only students or graduates of translation and interpreting, but also interpreters already working in the field who feel that they could benefit from training as they did not receive any when accessing the profession. It is also aimed at healthcare students or professionals who would like to work as healthcare interpreters, but in this case, some extra initial classes on interpreting would be included. The idea is to cover the gap in training and, in the future, to get this training recognized, as is the case in other countries where medical interpreting is more developed, such as the United Kingdom and the United States (Mikkelson 2020).

3.2. Italy

In Italy, universities and SSMLs (*Scuole Superiori per Mediatori Linguistici* [Linguistic Mediation Schools]) offer a large number of degrees in interpreting and translation or cultural/intercultural mediation, but no courses are specifically devoted to medical interpreting, which is sometimes taught in the form of a module within dialogue interpreting courses at the MA level. Some medical interpreting courses are offered by universities as extracurricular courses (*Alta Formazione*) and some private courses are offered, but it is difficult to obtain details about these.

The language combinations offered both by universities and private courses usually meet the needs of tourism and business, but do not meet the real needs of migrants and speakers of minority languages (see Chapter 2). According to Istat (*Istituto Nazionale di Statistica* 2019), Romanian is the largest linguistic community in Italy, followed by Arabic (including all regional varieties), Albanian, Spanish (mostly Latin American varieties), Chinese, Russian, Ukrainian, French, Serbian, Croatian, Polish, English, Bengali, Filipino, Sinhalese and others. The needs of these communities are often met by cultural/intercultural mediators with limited or no training in interpreting techniques and ethics, but who often share the same cultural background of the patients they are called on to assist in healthcare settings. Intercultural mediators are trained in courses totalling 450–600 hours organized and/or funded by regional authorities (*Regioni*), whose content aims to provide cultural/intercultural mediators with a basic knowledge of Italian legislation, some notions on the Italian healthcare system (*Servizio Sanitario Nazionale, SSN*) and basic cultural knowledge. These courses do not offer any training in interpreting skills or medical terminology.

During the four focus groups carried out by the ReACTMe Italian team (see Chapter 2), the interviewees (trainers, interpreters, cultural/intercultural mediators) were asked to suggest improvements to medical interpreting training, and they mentioned internships in hospitals and clinics for medical interpreting students, roleplays with healthcare professionals, the importance of debriefing and psychological support for interpreters and cultural/intercultural mediators.

3.3. Romania

In Romania, interpreting training programmes do not focus on medical interpreting *per se*. While there is a wide range of BA programmes and two MA programmes that train interpreters, there are no programmes that specifically train interpreters to work in healthcare contexts.

To fill this gap, Universitatea Babeș-Bolyai (UBB) is considering using the experience gained in the ReACTMe project to set up an elective training module for translation and interpreting students. The objective will be to target students with an interest in translation and interpretation and offer them specific training, especially in the areas that are more relevant to healthcare: medical terminology (anatomy, pathology), the ability to prepare and build terminological glossaries for various medical specialities, ethical issues regarding the relationship with both patients and medical staff, the ability to cope with vicarious trauma, etc. Healthcare staff or students should be invited to participate in the training programmes. Trainers specialized in medical terminology from the Universitatea de Medicină și Farmacie Iuliu Hațieganu, one of the partners of the ReACTMe project, will work together with trainers specialized in interpreting. Offered within an elective course, the classes would be open to students enrolled in BA and MA programmes within the Faculty of Letters. Another possibility currently envisaged is to offer a short-term training course (possibly a summer school) for freelance interpreters who want to acquire the necessary skills to better cope with the specificities of the healthcare context.

If successful, the programme could be advertised at a national level, as UBB is part of the Universitaria Consortium, a national body that comprises nine of the most important universities in Romania, all of them already offering BA and MA programmes in interpreting and/or translation. Since the consortium allows (at least in theory) the creation of common training programmes, a national training programme might also be a solution.

In Cluj-Napoca, an internship for interpreting and translation students could also address the specificities of working as a medical interpreter and provide the necessary experience in the field. UBB and teaching hospitals should sign protocols regarding the specific conditions of such internships, which would allow students to be exposed, under the supervision of both interpreting trainers and medical staff, to real-life situations.

Future training initiatives for medical interpreters in Romania should also target people with less common language combinations, which are taught to a lesser extent (if any) at university level, but which are needed in the healthcare context, such as Ukrainian (especially as a result of the recent refugee crisis), Turkish, Arabic, Urdu, Vietnamese and Nepalese. As seen in Chapter 1, English or French tend to be used as the *lingua franca* in medical contexts. However, the insufficient language level of some patients might lead to errors in communication.

Apart from these national initiatives, given the recent creation of a *Blended Intensive Programme* (BIP, <https://wikis.ec.europa.eu/pages/viewpage.action?pageId=48759218>) within the Erasmus+ framework, an international training programme might be a solution as it could aggregate know-how and specialized trainers available at a European level. A BIP is a short-term training programme offered jointly by at least three European universities, which must have a virtual component. The programme offers short-term mobilities for students and teachers and allows more flexibility as far as the courses are concerned, as students do not attend existing classes. Teachers can propose courses that are more relevant to the training even if they are not currently taught at their university. A BIP for medical interpreting would help the professionalization of future interpreters in this specific field as it would focus on particular topics relevant for healthcare contexts.

4. Recognition

As mentioned above, recognition is another key issue in the professionalization of any activity. However, it is important to differentiate between recognition by healthcare professionals (HCPs) and recognition by authorities as a profession that needs certification and accreditation.

As stated by Tomassini et al. (2022: 291), 'there is no specific national legislation regulating medical interpreting, nor specific references to medical interpreters, in either national or regional legislation in any of the three countries involved in this study.'

4.1. Spain

In Spain, national legislation does not refer specifically to translators or interpreters in healthcare settings; legislation on patients' rights only states that patients should receive the information, so they understand it, but does not explicitly mention the right to have an interpreter. As a result, in most Spanish Autonomous Communities, it is up to the healthcare authorities to decide whether or not an interpreter has to be provided. As for recognition by HCPs, it is a matter of educating these professionals on the importance and advantages of using professional interpreters to ensure that they request that the relevant healthcare authorities provide professional interpreters. The ReACTMe project has addressed this issue with the organization of different workshops with healthcare students and professionals, in which various topics were covered, such as the importance of working with professional interpreters, how to recognize a professional interpreter, the role of HCPs in achieving good communication when using interpreters and other important aspects that contribute to smooth communication. Furthermore, the ReACTMe team has also prepared a set of multilingual guidelines for working with medical interpreters (see Annex).

4.2. Italy

In Italy, national legislation mainly refers to intercultural mediators, with no mention made of interpreters. Similarly, regional legislation, which governs the provision of medical interpreting services, only refers to intercultural mediators. The great confusion between these two professional figures also impacts the way interpreters are perceived by HCPs, who erroneously believe that interpreters only provide linguistic support while intercultural mediators also cover the cultural aspects of the communication. Clients and patients do not seem to perceive the distinction.

It would be extremely important to address this problem of double definition for the providers of interpreting services, who should be defined either by the term 'interpreters' or by the word 'intercultural mediators' according to the peculiarities of their training and of the services they offer. This would help HCPs and patients to better understand what kind of services they can expect from the professionals appointed.

The European norms ISO 21998:20 – ISO 21998:2022–7 Interpreting services – Healthcare interpreting – Requirements and recommendations also apply to Italy, but these norms seem to be unknown to most of the HCPs interviewed, who made no mention of it (see Chapter 1).

4.3. Romania

Legislation in Romania does not distinguish between translators and interpreters. In practice, this situation translates into an abnormality: the Ministry of Culture organizes an examination for those who want to become certified (<www.culturadata.ro/examen-traducatori>); following the results of a translation exam, candidates become certified translators *and* interpreters. Candidates who have successfully passed the examination for legal translation can apply for certification at the Ministry of Justice and become sworn translators and interpreters. This certification is particularly useful for those who want to work as legal interpreters and translators, as the Romanian legislation stipulates that people who do not speak the national language should have a certified translator or interpreter in their interactions with the representatives of the judicial system. A certified interpreter is also mandatory when foreign citizens need the services of a notary public. To become a certified translator and interpreter for a given language, the candidate must successfully pass the translation test from and into that language (e.g. English into Romanian and Romanian into English). Although this certification from the Ministry of Justice is mandatory only for future legal translators and interpreters, the Ministry of Culture organizes certification exams for several domains: agriculture, arts, chemistry, computer science, economics, electronics and telecommunications, geography, history, law, literature, mathematics, philosophy-religion, physics, sociology-political sciences, technical sciences, and medicine-pharmacy.

The current legislation should be modified and impose the same rules for medical interpreters as for legal interpreters and at least make this examination mandatory for those who want to work in the Romanian healthcare system. The existing examination for medical-pharmaceutical translation could at least make candidates familiarize themselves with the specific terminology and organization of the Romanian healthcare system. Granted, a translation exam does not verify the future interpreter's aptitudes for interpretation, but it would at least set a minimum standard in a chaotic market. Additional specific training for interpreting skills, ethics and vicarious trauma could be offered in the training module offered by UBB and/or other HEIs. Ideally, the current legislation should be modified so as to clearly distinguish between translators and interpreters and, therefore, impose different certifications and examinations for both professions and set a rigorous national standard for medical interpreters.

5. The role of professional associations

Professional associations play a key role in developing professionalization, especially in unregulated professions where access criteria are not clear and where the role of professionals is not understood in the same way by all parties. As Mikkelson (1996: 83), citing Tseng (1992: 48–49), indicates,

> professionals can really work collectively with their colleagues to exert their influence over their job description and the behaviour of their colleagues, control admission into their circle and appeal to clients and the public for recognition of the profession. The power and achievements of the association strengthen the commitment of members to the course they are pursuing.

Professional associations fulfil different roles in the development of the profession of interpreting. These professional associations usually offer access to training resources, and they also establish standards and ethical codes for their members. This helps professionals to perform their job following a series of norms that are compulsory for members. Nevertheless, the problem arises when there are no specific associations, as is the case in most European countries where medical interpreters usually belong to more generic associations.

In Spain, over the last few years, there has been a rise in the number of associations representing translators and interpreters. The requirements to join Spanish associations differ from one association to another and the associations also have different categories of members. There are very few specific associations exclusively for interpreters, mainly AIIC España (*Asociación Internacional de Intérpretes de Conferencias*, <https://espana.aiic.org>) and AICE (*Asociación de Intérpretes de Conferencia de España*, <www.aice-interpretes.com>). Additionally, there are different translators associations at a national level, such as APTIJ (*Asociación Profesional de Traductores e Intérpretes Judiciales y Jurados*, <https://aptij.es>), ASETRAD (*Asociación Española de Traductores, Correctores e Intérpretes*, <https://asetrad.org>), and TREMEDICA (*Asociación Internacional de Traductores y*

Redactores de Medicina y Ciencias Afines), as well as associations at a regional level. Most of these associations admit interpreters as members but are not specifically dedicated to medical interpreting. However, although associations may play an important role in developing the profession, as they can be interlocutors when defining training and access criteria, their role is merely to advise and try to defend the profession, but they cannot oblige non-members to comply with their deontological codes as it is not compulsory to belong to professional associations to work in this field. The current role of most associations is more related to the dissemination of information about the profession of translators and interpreters and to the organization of training activities.

The main interpreter and translator associations in Italy are AIIC Italia (*Associazione Internazionale di Interpreti di Conferenza*, <https://aiic-italia.it>), AITI (*Associazione Italiana Traduttori e Interpreti*, <https://aiti.org/it>), ANITI (*Associazione Nazionale Italiana Traduttori e Interpreti*, <www.aniti.it>), and ASSOINTERPRETI (*Associazione Nazionale Interpreti di Conferenza Professionisti*, <www.assointerpreti.it>). In the association websites, it is possible to select professionals by name, language combination and/or specialization (Medicine and Veterinary), but no additional filter, such as years of experience in the field of specialization, is available. However, there are no specific associations for medical interpreters as there are in other countries, for example, in the United States.

Nationally and regionally recognized medical interpreting associations are not present in Italy. Healthcare services in Italy are governed and provided at a regional level, and certification for intercultural mediators, who also obtain basic knowledge of legislation and the healthcare system during their training, takes place at regional level. National and regional associations of medical interpreters would greatly help the professionalization of this service, which requires different specific skills and training from those of conference interpreting.

While some aspects of interpreter training overlap, others are area specific, such as terminology and language, as well as different language registers that apply to healthcare professionals and patients. Communication between doctors and patients is very often asymmetrical and medical interpreters sometimes adapt the language register to the level of the interlocutors to make the message clear for all the parties involved in the communication.

In Romania, there are two professional associations, APIT (*Asociația Profesională a Interpreților și Traducătorilor*, <www.apit.ro>) and UNTAR (*Uniunea Națională a Traducătorilor și Interpreților din România*, <www.traduceri-notariale.ro>), but judging by their websites, neither appears to be particularly active. For instance, the last event organized by APIT was in 2018.

Created in 2019, a group of translation professionals from Cluj organizes the *TranslateCluj* series of conferences, which have included workshops and presentations for interpreters. In 2022, a session dedicated to interpretation helped raise awareness on medical interpreters and the specificities of the profession through a presentation of the ReACTMe project.

Once translation and interpreting professionals understand the importance of specific training for medical interpreters, it would be important for them to begin a series of presentations for the Romanian healthcare community, for instance, during medical conferences. Perhaps in this way healthcare staff and administrators would better understand the benefits of employing professional interpreters in hospitals and other medical facilities.

6. Working conditions and suggestions for improvement

Working conditions can vary depending on the situation (different hospital departments, medical practices, emergency departments, operating theatres, etc.), but preparation for the interpreting assignment remains crucial. On the one hand, the interpreter is called for a previously programmed appointment. In this case, the interpreter, after being informed of the topic, must research the characteristics and consequences of the disease/procedure involved in the assignment. The relevant terminology must be studied, and a glossary prepared in both languages. On the other hand, there are emergency situations, as is usually the case in the emergency department, which require the skills of an interpreter trained to work in such a scenario, without preparing the relevant terminology and glossary.

Even in emergency situations, briefing is an essential element for interpreters as it allows them to obtain information about the context and the patient, which will be very useful for them when interpreting. Without the context, an interpreter does not know what to expect from the communicative situation.

In Spain, working conditions are not homogeneous for all medical interpreters but depend on the type of contract. In private hospitals, there are sometimes in-house interpreters who also perform different administrative tasks. In public hospitals, interpreting services are usually outsourced to agencies that provide interpreters on demand. In some cases, there are interpreters who work with a fixed shift in hospitals but are employed by external companies. In the case of interpreters on demand, they are frequently freelance interpreters, and have to pay their own social security costs and other job-related expenses. They are usually paid on an hourly basis, and the rate depends greatly on the individual translation and interpreting company. Companies providing these services are selected after a public call, and in order to obtain these contracts, some companies reduce the price that the administration will have to pay for the interpreting services. This means that the company then needs to get interpreters to work for very low rates of pay, which can influence the quality of interpreting services because professional interpreters will refuse to work under such conditions. Companies, therefore, sometimes use 'interpreters' without any kind of training who are considered interpreters merely because they speak two languages. In the case of remote interpreting, the most widely used mode is telephone interpreting. In these cases, interpreters are usually paid per minute. As there is free market by law, associations cannot recommend rates, so the rate paid will greatly depend on the negotiations between the company and the interpreter. In cases where the professional interpreter is hired directly by the patient, there are no recommended rates, so interpreters have to negotiate prices directly with the patient.

In Italy, medical interpreting is not recognized as a profession *per se*, but more as a specialization within the profession, that is, interpreters choose to specialize in medical interpreting. Furthermore, as previously explained, there are two professional figures covering the need to overcome linguistic barriers: interpreters and (inter)cultural mediators. The latter are mostly used for the communication with native speakers of minority languages and their training is often not at university level (see Section 3 on Training). As stated by Baraldi and Gavioli (2016: 33), 'intercultural mediators do not necessarily have a professional training in interpreting, they are, however, preferred to professional interpreters in that they are considered more competent in mediating the possibly different perspectives of healthcare providers and migrant patients.'

When medical interpreters or cultural/intercultural mediators are not available, ad hoc interpreters are used; these tend to be nurses, doctors or hospital employees who happen to speak the other language, or family members or friends of the patient, sometimes even children. This situation implies many risks because people who have not received any training in interpreting skills or medical terminology only translate what they hear, sometimes not even understanding it and often omitting or adding content. Moreover, the emotional burden in the case of conveying bad news during interpreting could even lead ad hoc interpreters to omit or change the information in order not to scare or worry their family members or friends. This is particularly true when children are involved in interpreting for their parents. This practice should always be discouraged because healthcare professionals and patients are not aware of the risks and issues involved.

In Italy, payment and rates mainly depend on the client assigning the professional. Most hospitals make use of cooperatives and NGOs to provide the interpreting services and rates can vary greatly. When the assignment is direct (i.e. the patient or hospital department directly assigns a freelance interpreter), there is room for negotiation.

Although the COVID-19 pandemic affected all countries and continents, Italy was the first European country to be hit by the pandemic and to experience lockdown. During this period, interpreting changed from face-to-face to remote interpreting and many professionals, above all senior interpreters, had to adapt to new technologies and methods for providing their services. According to the results of an online survey submitted to medical interpreters/cultural mediators from all over Italy between November 2020 and January 2021,

> [T]he pandemic has negatively affected the provision of medical interpreting/cultural mediation services with remote communication only partially making up for the lack of onsite language support and creating new challenges for both interpreters/cultural mediators and healthcare professionals. (Bernardi and Gnani 2022: 54)

As for the duration of the interpreting service, it often depends on the type of assignment and the hospital department in which it takes place. A few hospitals in Italy have internal interpreting services where the professionals are employees who work on a shift basis, while other facilities appoint a freelancer when they need to overcome language barriers and only for the service and the language combination needed.

Professional Indemnity Insurance (PII) is not compulsory in Italy, but it is recommended by some major professional associations such as AITI (2022: online), which also offers 'particularly advantageous professional insurance and health insurance policies'. PII can help medical interpreters in cases of errors during interpreting.

As far as Romania is concerned, the working conditions (rates, labour contract, working hours, preparation, etc.) are discussed using legal translation and interpreting as a point of reference, as it is the only domain regulated by current legislation. There are standard rates within the country for legal translators and interpreters, but they are very low. According to the 2907/C/2340/2020 Order of the Ministry of Justice, sworn translators and interpreters working for public institutions belonging to the Romanian judicial system should be paid 30.91 lei/hour (roughly 6.30 euros) for interpretation and 44.82 lei/page (a little over 9 euros) for translation. For Asian languages the rates are double, and for simultaneous interpretation, regardless of language combination, rates are double as well. It is important to mention that these rates are subject to tax, so an interpreter with English or French earns around 4 euros per hour when working for Romanian judicial institutions.

There are no standard rates for medical interpreting, as the profession is completely unregulated in Romania, but one may safely assume that these official fees may be used in the healthcare system, especially when public hospitals or clinics have to pay. When the patient himself/herself hires an interpreter, we can assume that the interpreter can negotiate higher rates, as one interpreter confirmed during the focus groups carried out within the

ReACTMe project. Nonetheless, the low rates paid by the public sector is a demotivating factor for both current professional interpreters and future ones. In most cases, private agencies of freelance translators and interpreters provide medical interpreting services, but their rates are not public, so we may assume that they are negotiated before the signing of each contract.

According to the focus groups with Romanian professional interpreters conducted in the ReACTMe project, availability and confidentiality clauses are included in interpreters' contracts. According to one of the participants, who is a freelance interpreter and has a contract with a hospital, in the first draft of the contract it was stipulated that the interpreter should arrive within ten minutes of being called by the hospital. During the negotiations, the clause was changed to two hours when the interpreter is available. As far as preparation is concerned, there is no available data for medical interpreting, but we can assume that professional interpreters who collaborate with hospitals feel the need to prepare carefully before an assignment. However, we do not have any information about the briefing practices in this context and we consider that more awareness-raising campaigns are necessary in healthcare institutions, as medical staff or medical administrators may not yet understand the importance of a detailed briefing before working with interpreters.

To sum up, working conditions for Romanian interpreters in general, and for medical interpreters in particular, need improvement or standardization. Higher rates would make the profession more appealing for younger interpreters, and a clear set of standards regarding working hours, availability, and briefing would have a positive impact on quality.

As this volume shows, there is still room for improvement in the situation of medical interpreting and interesting suggestions arose during the focus groups organized with professional interpreters and trainers.

Some participants commented on the importance of having first aid courses at the outset of training or as a prerequisite (both as a coping test and as terminological and procedural preparation). Internships are also considered a good opportunity before becoming a full professional. Recognition from other professionals is crucial. This recognition could be reflected in the certification of the course by the National Board of Physicians and finally, some of them also mentioned to adopt some of the accreditation procedures and training methods used for legal interpreters and adapt them to the needs of the interpreting in the medical field.

In the case of training, it is important to develop a good definition of the target audience: are we addressing interpreting/translation students or graduates, medical students, nurses? Depending on the target audience, a devoted language register should be used and taught. However, different target audiences could be also combined using different pedagogical materials depending on the background of the students.

Professionalizing medical interpreting also means including different aspects that are not sufficiently considered in Italy, Spain and Romania during formal training at university level. One of these is interpreting for children. It is often assumed that participants in the communicative events are adults, but this is not always the case. In healthcare settings, interpreting for children can be necessary and requires a specific approach. Wadensjö (1998) describes a situation in which a 7-year-old girl has to undergo a blood test and is scared. According to the scholar, the interpreter did not assume the role that she usually does in the presence of adults; she did not in fact maintain a detached role, thereby breaking one of the basic rules of an interpreter's code of ethics. Rather, as Wadensjö (ibid.) asserts, she took on the guise of a kindly adult, speaking in a soft tone of voice throughout the encounter and reassuring the child about the blood-drawing. As can be seen from the dialogue reported by the author, the interpreter even started a private conversation with the child just as the needle was being inserted. All these actions are the result of autonomous decisions by the interpreter and are subject to very specific motivations. As all interpreters working for children know very well, it is often impossible to maintain a completely detached and cold role with the child if the communicative act is to be successful. In the situation described by Wadensjö (ibid.), the interpreter's attitude of greater emotional involvement does not correspond to a lack of neutrality. She remains neutral with respect to the parties, as all actions taken autonomously have the dual purpose of calming the child and helping to proceed with the objective of the meeting, namely collecting the blood sample. It is worth noticing that the child only speaks when her mother asks her a question, an attitude that is very common in children because they only trust the people they know they can rely on. Reflecting on the role of the child (especially at a very young age) in interpreter-mediated communication, Wadensjö (ibid.: 185) points out that he/she plays a very flexible role in the communicative event, stating that 'a child can abruptly be transformed/transform her- or himself from a person talked and listened to, into an object talked about and vice versa'. Finally, she adds that 'the person who speaks least appears to be the one who exercises the greatest influence on the interpreter's role performance' (ibid.).

When interpreting for children in particular, briefing plays an essential role and should be scheduled whenever conditions allow it. During briefing, interpreters can ask questions to children, parents and healthcare professionals, gathering important information.

At the beginning of the interview with the child, it is crucial that there is a clear definition of roles between the parties. The introduction should be formulated in a language that is appropriate to the age and cognitive development of the child. It must be clear and should involve simple vocabulary. Regarding the presentation of oneself and one's role, the Phoenix Children's Hospital (cited in Amato 2021) recommends using a presentation of the type suggested below:

> Hi! I am the interpreter.
> When someone says something in English, I repeat in Spanish.
> When someone says something in Spanish, I repeat in English.

Students, as well as healthcare professionals, should be made aware of the difference between interpreting for adults and for children, and all these aspects should be included in medical interpreting training using roleplays to practise it. The comparison between interpreting for children and interpreting for adults, such as the one offered by the Phoenix Children's Hospital (cited in Amato 2021), could help students to have an overview of the main differences that exist in communication and interaction with the two groups.

Another aspect that should be considered during training is medical interpreting for mental health settings, which would deserve separate training, perhaps in the form of a dedicated module. Doherty et al. (2010) have investigated the impact that interpreting for clients with mental health problems had on 157 surveyed interpreters contracted by Glasgow

Translating and Interpreting Services in the UK. The responses of eighteen interpreters were analysed and revealed that all the interpreters had been emotionally affected to varying degrees by the interpreting assignment, some of them mentioning feelings of anger, sadness, hopelessness and powerlessness after their job. During training it is very important to make students aware of this risk, as well as of the risk of vicarious trauma when working with victims of violence.

Working as a medical interpreter implies many responsibilities, time pressure due to emergency and emotional burden which could sometimes lead to errors during the assignment. It is suggested and recommended to enter a professional indemnity insurance (PII), even though it is very expensive in some countries.

7. Conclusions

As we have seen in this chapter, there is still a long way to go to reach full professionalization of medical interpreting in Spain, Italy and Romania. However, these three countries involved in the ReACTMe project are beginning to go in the right direction. It is necessary to guarantee that medical interpreting services are provided to a high standard and, to achieve that, training is crucial. If interpreters are trained, they will undoubtedly do a better job, but recognition is also very important to attract good interpreters to medical interpreting. This recognition should be linked to attractive rates for interpreting jobs; if interpreters are trained and recognized by other professionals, but this is not reflected in their pay, the job will not attract professional interpreters.

The pandemic has shown that healthcare can save lives, but that communication is also crucial in these situations. The right of an individual to access medical care/healthcare services is included in Article 25-1 of the Universal Declaration of Human Rights (UDHR), which states: 'Everyone has the right to a standard of living adequate for the health and well-being of himself and of his family, including food, clothing, housing and *medical care* and necessary social services, and the right to security in the event of unemployment, sickness, disability, widowhood, old age or other lack of livelihood in circumstances beyond his control.' Nevertheless, language barriers can cause disparities in accessing adequate and high-quality healthcare services. These barriers can be overcome by appointing medical interpreters who are equipped to professionally interpret the communication between patients and healthcare professionals. If the profession of medical interpreting is not adequately recognized in terms of training, working conditions and rates, it will be difficult to discuss its professionalization, which could result in a one-way effort on the part of interpreters. Moreover, professional associations at national and regional level should consider creating a special list of medical interpreters specifically trained to work in healthcare settings.

This chapter has suggested some urgent improvements to be made in Spain, Italy, and Romania. The suggestions are not exhaustive, but their implementation would be a good start in the professionalization of medical interpreting in the three countries.

Bibliography

Amato, Amalia & Gabriele Mack. 2021. 'The best interest of the child in interpreter-mediated interviews. Researching children's point of view', *inTRAlinea* 23. http://www.intralinea.org/archive/article/2539

Baraldi, Claudio, and Laura Gavioli. 2016. 'On professional and non-professional interpreting in healthcare services: The case of intercultural mediators', *European Journal of Applied Linguistics* 4(1), 33–51.

Bernardi, Eleonora, and Francesca Gnani. 2022. 'The impact of the COVID-19 pandemic on medical interpreters/cultural mediators in Italy', *FITISPOS International Journal* 9(1), 54–77. <https://fitisposij.web.uah.es/OJS/index.php/fitispos/article/view/307>.

Doherty, Sharon M., Anna M. MacIntyre, and Tara Wyne. 2010. 'How does it feel for you? The emotional impact and specific challenges of mental health interpreting', *Mental Health Review Journal* 15(3), 31–44.

Downing, Bruce, and Karin Ruschke. 2012. 'Professionalizing healthcare interpreting between spoken languages', in Laurie Swabey and Karen Malcolm (eds), *In Our*

Hands: Educating Healthcare Interpreters. Washington: Gallaudet University Press, 209–228.

Hale, Sandra. 2007. *Community Interpreting*. Basingstoke: Palgrave Macmillan.

Mikkelson, Holly. 1996. 'The professionalization of community interpreting', in M. Jérôme-O'Keeffe (ed.), *Global Vision: Proceedings of the 37th Annual Conference of the American Translators Association*. Alexandria, VA: American Translators Association, 77–89.

Pena-Díaz, Carmen. 2018. 'Ethics in theory and practice in Spanish healthcare community interpreting', *MonTI* 10, 93–115.

Tomassini, Elena, Almudena Nevado Llopis, Ana Isabel Foulquié Rubio, Christopher Garwood, Alina Andreica, and Alina Pelea. 2002. 'Medical interpreting in Spain, Italy and Romania: A comparative study', in Maria Pilar, Castillo Bernal, and Marta Estévez Grossi (eds), *Translation, Mediation and Accessibility for Linguistic Minorities*. Berlin: Frank & Time, 287–301.

Tseng, Joseph. 1992. *Interpreting as an Emerging Profession in Taiwan – A Sociological Model*. Unpublished Master's Thesis, Taiwan: Fu Jen Catholic University.

Wadensjö, Cecilia. 1998. *Interpreting as Interaction*. New York: Longman.

ELEONORA BERNARDI AND LINDSEY BRUTON

4 Training Resources and Methodologies for Medical Interpreters

1. Introduction

In this chapter dedicated to the ReACTMe project we focus on which resources and methodologies can best be applied to the training of medical interpreters. This was one of the first questions the research teams in the project addressed, as two of the project's goals were to design a curriculum to train medical interpreters to be implemented after the funding period, and to train trainers and university students both at undergraduate and postgraduate level.

Although medical interpreting training has a history, especially in Scandinavian and Anglo-Saxon countries, deciding which resources could best be used to train medical interpreters was not an easy task, requiring the project's research teams to carry out an in-depth review of existing training programmes and online resource compilations available. Despite the abundance of resources on the internet, many were not freely accessible and those that were had to be selected, ranked and evaluated. The risk, otherwise, as colleagues reading this are probably aware, would have been that of creating a patchwork of resources that had no consistency, or progression and were not linked to students' level and pedagogical goals. Owing to this lack of coherently organized resources, many trainers continue to create resources of their own, especially roleplays, which is undoubtedly time-consuming and challenging.

In an attempt to counter this problem, the ReACTMe research teams located accessible online and open-access resources both in the official languages of the project (English, Spanish, Italian and Romanian) and, when available, in other languages that could be useful for the acquisition and development of competences necessary for interpreting in healthcare settings. These resources were first analysed and evaluated by the project partners and catalogued using the system of competences that will be explained in Section 2.1., later in this chapter. The idea was to provide a set of reliable training resources that could be used by learners for autonomous study, by trainers who might want to extend and improve the resources they use in class and by professional interpreters wanting to specialize in medical interpreting or needing to develop one specific competence. In addition to cataloguing existing resources, the ReACTMe researchers also decided to create original resources for training medical interpreters, expressly to fill gaps identified in the mapping of existing resources. These took the form of roleplays, terminological exercises, case studies and glossaries available on the ReACTMe training platform.

Parallelly, the project members also investigated what the best methods to teach medical interpreting were, based on the literature available on this topic and their experience as medical interpreters and trainers of interpreters. The methods selected, which cover those most widely used, but are by no means all-inclusive, are those that the literature and experience recognized as most useful in the training of medical interpreters and which were also identified as such in the training events organized by the project, according to feedback received from trainers and trainees.

In this chapter we will therefore describe the selection process, and organization of the resources that proved most effective for teaching medical interpreters catalogued by the ReACTMe project (Section 2.1), as well as the original resources created and available on the project's learning platform (Section 2.2). We will then briefly present the training methods we identified as most operative and the rationale behind their use (Section 3). We conclude by reflecting on the changing face of education and how we believe that the resources available on the ReACTMe platform and the Key elements to be considered when designing a course for medical interpreters (presented in Chapter 5 of this volume) may contribute to progress in this field.

2. Resources

Research carried out in the year 1 of the ReACTMe project (2019–2020) showed that there is a lack of resources available to teach medical interpreting online, both for trainees who would like to improve their skills both in class and autonomously online, and for trainers, who are often obliged to develop their own materials, at great cost in terms of both time and energy, and consequently keep them for themselves. ReACTMe partners therefore decided that offering some of these resources on its learning platform would be helpful for both trainers and trainees and decided to offer (a) a collection of existing training resources, described in Section 2.1, and (b) original training material and resources, discussed in Section 2.2 of this chapter, including a multilingual glossary organized according to medical specialities.

2.1. *The cataloguing of existing resources*

For the creation of a database of existing resources for teaching and learning medical interpreting, during 2020 and 2021, the project partners undertook research to select and describe available resources in English, and the languages of the project partners (Spanish, Italian and Romanian), but it also included resources in French and German in addition to languages of more limited diffusion.

To categorize and classify these resources, the literature was reviewed to establish the main competences considered necessary for effective interpreting in healthcare settings. Seven competences were identified: instrumental and professional, communicative and textual, cultural and intercultural, thematic, interpersonal, strategic and psychophysiological. The nomenclature of these competences varies among authors but their meanings and the skills they encompass are, in general, very similar. For example, the communicative and textual competence is called linguistic and communicative competence by Pöchhacker (2004) and Sawyer (2004) and is simply denominated linguistic competence by Angelelli (2019).

Similarly, what is called thematic competence in the ReACTMe project is denominated extralinguistic competence by some authors (PACTE 2001).

The areas covered by each competence in the ReACTMe project, as explained by Nevado Llopis and Foulquié Rubio (2022: 1680–1693), are the following:

- Instrumental and professional competence refers to three areas of practice: the effective and appropriate use of tools and resources; the management of a professional career in terms of certification and membership in professional bodies; and adherence to the ethical and deontological norms of the profession.
- Communicative and textual competence alludes to what others call linguistic competence. It includes aspects relating to language, such as knowledge of medical terminology, dialects, registers varieties of language and turn-taking norms in medical settings. In addition, it covers the application of this knowledge to real-life contexts.
- Cultural and intercultural competence includes knowledge of cultural and sociocultural patterns, specifically those relating to health and medicine in addition to knowledge of demographics, migration and the way in which cultural values may affect communication.
- Thematic competence encompasses extralinguistic knowledge: knowledge of the health system that the interpreter is working within and specialist medical knowledge in particular fields. It also presupposes the knowledge of the structure of healthcare services, professional categories, procedures and protocols followed, etc.
- Interpersonal competence includes many aspects of mediation, such as critical thinking, ethical commitment, the ability to work in a team, to arbitrate, resolve conflicts and justify decisions taken.
- Strategic competence covers the knowledge and skills necessary to successfully carry out the interpretation techniques required in the medical field in both face-to-face and online encounters: liaison

interpreting, consecutive interpreting, note-taking, sight translation and occasionally simultaneous interpreting.
- Psychophysiological competence refers to skills such as concentration, memory, and the capacity for analysis and reformulation as well as the ability to manage stress and distance oneself from emotionally distressing situations.

It goes without saying that these competences are closely connected and interwoven in the work of a professional medical interpreter and that the development of one competence directly influences the development of others: for example, the strategic competence, which requires the interpreter to master the interpreting techniques necessary to carry out the task, such as note-taking and active listening, will necessarily also help them develop communicative and interpersonal competences, given that the interaction between the participants in a medical interpreting event is eminently social in nature.

The resources identified, evaluated and checked by the project teams had, therefore, to contribute to the development of one or more of these competences in addition to being online, open access, and in the languages of the project (Spanish, Italian, Romanian or English) or any other language. Once selected and organized according to the competences outlined above, the resources compilation was made available on the ReACTMe learning platform under the heading ReACTMe Training Resources Compilation. At present, more than 150 resources have been indexed on the ReACTMe database with certain resources appearing under more than one competence heading owing to the overlap in competence development mentioned above. Resources are more abundant for the instrumental and professional, communicative and textual and the thematic competences and there are considerably more resources available in English and, to a lesser extent, in Spanish, than in the other languages present in the database. This lack of resources in certain areas in other languages was addressed to an extent with the creation of original materials also available on the ReACTMe learning platform, which we hope will continue to be expanded in the future.

Users can filter the resources in the Training Resources Compilation by language and by competence and will obtain a list of all resources for that language and competence as we can see in the example in Figure 4.1, where, for example, resources to develop cultural & intercultural competence in English are shown.

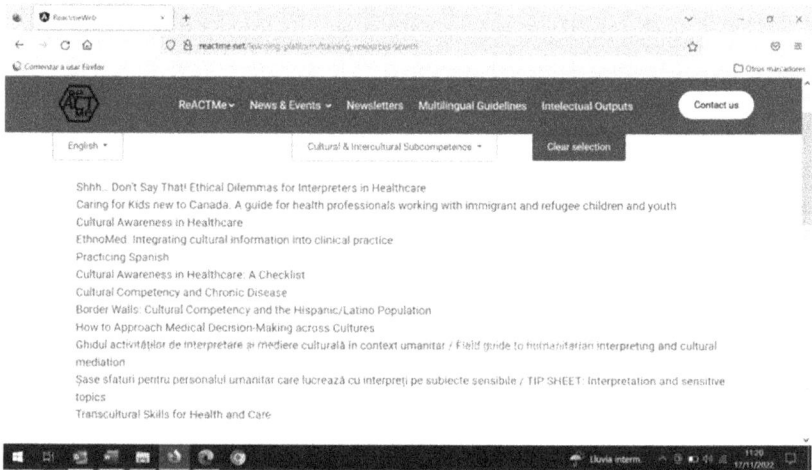

Figure 4.1. ReACTMe learning platform: English resources for the development of cultural and intercultural competences

After the resource has been selected, by clicking on it, it is possible to visualize information for each resource which includes its title, languages used, main and other competences to be developed, a link to the resource, a brief description of contents and function and use, that is, whether the resource is best suited to face-to-face training or autonomous study. We can see an example of the 'index card' available for each resource in Figure 4.2, which shows the information available for the resource titled 'Shh… Don't say that! Ethical dilemmas for interpreters in healthcare'.

We consider that the resources collection is quite extensive, as it covers competences that have often been neglected in interpreters' training (Bancroft et al. 2015) such as the psychophysiological competence, which features resources related to training for trauma avoidance and stress management for medical interpreters, for example. However, we hope that in addition to being a go-to place for trainers and learners, the platform can also be a starting point for a bank of resources that can be extended in the

Training Resources and Methodologies 133

existing and other languages and updated in the future, perhaps with the help of other universities and projects.

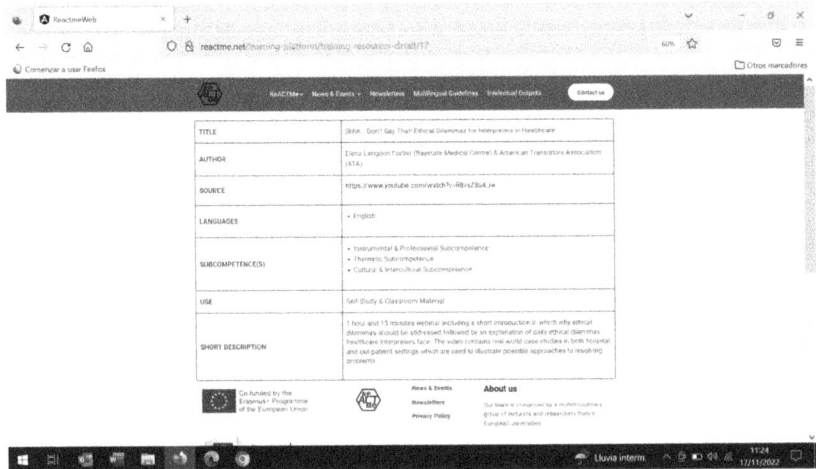

Figure 4.2. ReACTMe platform: example of training resources 'index card'

2.2. *The creation of original resources*

Although the Training Resources Compilation comprised a useful collection of tools and tasks for medical interpreter training, our state-of-the-art analysis of resources and research carried out in year 1 of the project pointed to a lack of appropriate resources in certain areas. Resources that we found to be lacking were terminological exercises developed specifically for interpreters, case studies and, most importantly, roleplays, which, as we will see in Section 3 of this chapter, have long been the staple of dialogue interpreter training. To meet this need, the project developed a second bank of resources, this time original ones, created expressly by ReACTMe team members with the help of language trainers and healthcare professionals, to train medical interpreters. These are the ReACTMe Training Resources, available on the project's learning platform, which feature five types of original resources: terminological exercises, roleplays, case studies, didactic units and a multilingual glossary. The resources have been conceived of for both self-study or asynchronous learning, as in the case of terminological exercises, for example, and for use in class under the guidance of a trainer, as with case studies and roleplays. The materials created are described below.

The platform features ten original case studies, all in English, which usually begin with a profile of the patient and a brief description of the other participants involved, continue with an overview of the context and problematic situation and then offer a series of questions about how the interpreter should respond to challenges arising in this situation. Sometimes imagined, sometimes mirroring real events in medical interpreting as experienced by ReACTMe project members, our case study exercises are suitable for both online and face-to-face training sessions but require an environment where discussion is possible among trainees and trainers and are more suitable for trainees who do have some level of awareness and maturity, for example, MA students.

The roleplay section proposes dialogues in combinations of two languages (English–Spanish; English–Italian; English–Romanian; Spanish–Romanian; Italian–Romanian) between a patient and a specialist from different medical domains: cardiology (two roleplays), emergency room (one roleplay), orthopaedic surgery and orthopaedics (three roleplays), paediatrics (one roleplay), sleep clinic (one roleplay), oncology (one roleplay), primary care (one roleplay) and gynaecology (one roleplay) for a total of eleven roleplays in different language combinations. The level of difficulty is medium, as these roleplays were conceived to be used with learners in higher education who have either been studying medicine/nursing or interpreting, but they can be calibrated by each trainer to match specific needs and levels. The difficulty of the roleplays can be increased, and other skills can be practised by including, for example, patient consent forms or patient histories to be sight translated. Although these roleplay exercises can and have been employed online – as was done during the ReACTMe First Intensive Programme for Higher Education Learners in July 2021 – it would be preferable to conduct them face-to-face to take full advantage of the interaction between all participants involved (doctor/patient/other people/interpreter).

Terminological exercises were created for cardiology, gynaecology, oncology, ophthalmology, orthopaedics, pharmacology and toxicology, surgery, and COVID-19.[1] According to expert opinion and previous research, these areas were identified as being the most useful and frequently encountered in medical interpreting in the countries involved in the project. The exercises are offered in English, Italian, Spanish and Romanian to help trainees develop an interlanguage competence for each field as will be further explained in Section 3.6. Exercises feature different types of texts but, in general, they were selected and created so that specialized vocabulary is contextualized, and content and description of the terms introduced is provided to enrich students' general knowledge about the respective medical fields. Exercises are presented in a manner that leads students to discover and understand specialized vocabulary and gain confidence in the use of specialized lexis when confronted with it in interpreting activities. Filling in the blanks, completing the missing form of words, matching the word with the definition, and finding the common name for some medical terms are just some of the tasks that students can be asked to complete in asynchronous work, although these exercises could also be done in class, in small groups that later report and discuss their terminological choices. Each exercise has an answer key at the end so that students can check their answers autonomously and redo those that they consider more difficult, gaining speed in completing the tasks.

Additionally, the platform features five didactic units, each of which includes terminology exercises, a roleplay and a case study as well as an introduction briefly outlining the topic, the ethical challenges the interpreter will face, and the goals and outcomes of the learning process. These didactic units were developed during the ReACTMe Short-Term Staff Training Event for trainers held in January 2021 online, instead of in Cluj-Napoca, Romania, in 2020 due to the COVID-19 pandemic. The training event gathered university translation, interpreting or foreign language

---

1   With medicine being a vast field, with many subfields of specialization, we focused on those that were, according to the authors experience as medical interpreters and medical interpreting trainers and researchers, most frequently worked in, in addition to being within the project members' fields of specialization.

lecturers from the six participating universities, who were asked to develop training resources together following a set of guidelines and input provided by trainers. The resulting didactic units were later verified, corrected and standardized by the project members.

Finally, among the ReACTMe original training resources there is also a multilingual glossary to support interpreters in getting to know medical concepts and terms and to work with as a user-friendly resource when in doubt on the job. As Medicine is a vast field, with several macro fields and subfields, we narrowed our focus to eight specialties: cardiology, surgery, COVID-19, pharmacology and toxicology, oncology, gynaecology, ophthalmology, and orthopaedics with a total of 564 items.[2] Some of these, such as COVID-19, pharmacology and oncology, were very present while the project was being developed, while others, like cardiology, orthopaedics, and gynaecology, represent some of the most frequent contexts in which medical interpreters work, for example, a tourist breaking a leg or a migrant woman accessing a pregnancy clinic.

The glossary was drafted by a team of healthcare students and professionals in one of the universities participating in this project, who selected and reviewed the terms in English. Once the glossary, or rather glossaries, were ready, they were translated into Italian, Romanian and Spanish by a translator and then reviewed by a healthcare professional, doctor or nurse, with a good knowledge of English and the local language (Italian, Romanian or Spanish).

Each glossary entry features the English term, a definition of the term and the definition source, and its translation to the three target languages. Definitions were included in all the languages because, as we have said, they help interpreters to learn not just the corresponding term in Italian, for example, for 'ablation', but also to understand what the procedure is about, which is especially important in medical interpreting. Definitions are also explanations; they offer the chance to learn synonyms or help paraphrase if the interpreter cannot find an equivalent in another language.

---

2   Seventy-three items for pharmacology, sixty for COVID-19, 156 for cardiology, forty-three for surgery, forty-eight for oncology, fifty-six for gynaecology, fifty for ophthalmology and seventy-eight for orthopaedics.

The ability to paraphrase and define has been proven to be a crucial skill in medical interpreting.

3. Methods and activities

In interpreter training, as in any type of training, methods are closely linked to and reflected in learning activities. Consequently, no reflection on resources was possible without parallelly defining the most suitable methods to train medical interpreters. As already explained in the introduction, without proper data to scientifically affirm that the methods used are the best in absolute terms, the project partners analysed the available literature for training medical interpreters and dialogue interpreters in general and tapped into their own experience as medical interpreters and trainers. The methods described here therefore do not pretend to represent the rule, nor are they an exhaustive list, but they are the ones that have proved most useful in the experience of this project and those that the trainers and trainees taking part in the ReACTMe training activities have most appreciated and found most effective. In this section we will present the main methods and activities used in the training of medical interpreters: case studies, monolingual videos, sight translation exercises, roleplays, written texts and terminological exercises. For each of these we will provide a brief description of the method and the theory behind it, explaining why we feel they are effective methods and/or activities and how they are used in the development of the seven competences identified for medical interpreters.

3.1. Case studies

Case studies as a pedagogic approach have long been used in higher education, initially developed by prestigious American universities in the fields of Business and Law and, more recently, in the context of healthcare. They are scenarios in the form of narratives describing a particular situation which must be analysed and resolved by learners (Herreid 2011). The approach requires learners to draw on existing theoretical knowledge, and with expert guidance, move towards a deeper understanding of complex situations and at the same time familiarize students with situations that might occur in real life and prepare them to have ethically correct reactions or to at least to reflect on the complexity of reality, which sometimes goes beyond the tenets of ethical guidelines. For example, they might present situations where an ethical dilemma arises, and the medical interpreter is called upon to make a decision like whether the interpreter should translate offensive statements, influence decisions, or omit sensitive explanations that could contribute to a better understanding of the message. The trainee knows that they should in theory remain impartial, but case studies can reveal that life is not always black or white and that difficult decisions must be taken.

The case study approach has been shown to increase student engagement and learning and the use of higher order thinking skills (Rybarczyk 2007), while other studies have proved that learners are more likely to be motivated and learn from complex, controversial cases that are relevant to their lives and learning (Bain 2004). Case studies can also be used to motivate learners to seek new knowledge and apply it to a specific, practical context. They can, therefore, teach students how to apply theory in practice but can also be used to induce theory from practice. In whatever way case studies are used, they have been shown to encourage the use of critical thinking and analysis, decision making, judgement and action. Some would argue that the use of case studies is more effective with students at postgraduate level who have more experience and knowledge to draw on, but the approach may be used too at undergraduate level in the hands of a skilled guide who can apply the relevant Socratic questioning to lead learners towards a deeper understanding of the case.

In the specific context of training medical interpreters, case studies often present an ethical dilemma or intercultural misunderstanding that might occur in interaction and as such are useful in the development of cultural and intercultural, interpersonal and psychophysiological competences.

For example, in the case study that we see in Figure 4.3, extracted from the ReACTMe learning platform, the parents of a 5-year-old Romanian boy are delivered a difficult diagnosis by a British doctor through an interpreter. The doctor uses very obscure and specific terminology, and the interpreter follows the doctor's register by offering a technical translation of the child's medical issue which the parents do not understand and, even worse, are under the impression that everything is fine. The student interpreter or trainee is asked here to decide what the interpreter/or themselves should do/have done in this case, if it is better to use a technical rather than a colloquial register, and what they would do when they realized that a serious misunderstanding has occurred.

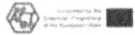

LEARNING PLATFORM- Case Study

CASE STUDY 8. MISUNDERSTANDING ABOUT THE GRAVITY OF THE DIAGNOSIS
(PAEDIATRICS)

PATIENT AND FAMILY PROFILE

A 5-year old boy comes to the hospital with his parents for the results of the tests he has undergone these last weeks. The family is Romanian, and they came to the UK after several months spent in Romanian hospitals to find out the cause of the boy's poor health. None of the three speaks English. Parents do not have a good level of medical education.

DESCRIPTION OF THE CASE STUDY

The parents are confident that British doctors will diagnose and treat their son correctly. Moreover, as the boy has been feeling better these last days, they are optimistic about today's appointment and expect to receive good news.
The doctor is very worried about the boy's health and considers it is best to inform them about the pessimistic prognosis in an indirect way, using medical terminology that obscures – from the parents' perspective – the truth. The interpreter chooses to be faithful to the doctor's choice and renders the information correctly both from the point of view of content and register. Parents are misled and seem to conclude that the doctor is control and knows how to treat the boy. They start smiling, thank the doctor for his help and say they will do whatever it takes to see their son healthy again. The doctor is puzzled by this reaction and looks at the interpreter doubtfully.

After having read the case study, answer the following questions:

1. Should the interpreter intervene and tell the doctor that, according to what she overheard, the parents do not seem to have understood that the situation is not improving?
2. Should the interpreter intervene by turning the doctor's euphemistic language into a more direct one? Can she avoid doing so without being too blunt?

Figure 4.3. Case study 8. Misunderstanding about the gravity of the diagnosis
Source: ReACTMe learning platform

This case study, as all other case studies on the learning platform, exemplifies the fact that medical interpreting does not only consist of listening, translating and speaking, but that it involves choices and decision making. Decisions that must be made in real time and which may not be covered by explicit ethical guidelines.

3.2. *(Monolingual) videos*

As a faithful or recreated reproduction of real-life experience, monolingual videos that can be found online have been mainly created to train medical professionals in the intricacies of medical communication. As such, they are an invaluable resource that in our setting allow learners to obtain a much fuller picture of a medical exchange between practitioner and patient than any written text can provide, especially if produced for students of Medicine or Nursing, as they offer realistic depictions of doctor-patient or nurse-patient encounters. If the videos are monolingual and feature 'real' unscripted examples of exchanges between healthcare providers and patients, the language will be much more natural than in a scripted roleplays, for example, with all the hesitations, repetitions, redundancies and unfinished sentences characteristic of natural speech, and the learner will have the chance to learn language in context and develop more natural language solutions. This type of video can also be used to illustrate concepts, to provide exposure to real medical communication which has its rules and phases and can help the interpreters prepare for the different stages of a medical encounter, know their purpose, recurring language and aims.

Monolingual videos can also be used to reflect on the positioning of participants in an exchange and on their body language, on their attitudes and use of language, and, as Garwood and Tomassini state in Chapters 5 and 6 of this volume, monolingual videos help trainees with the pronunciation of terms and towards a deeper understanding of terminology.

Bilingual or multilingual videos, that is, videos showing interactions between the interpreter, and a healthcare provider and patient who do not share the same language can also be used in class: they offer some of the advantages of monolingual videos, with the additional opportunity to listen to and analyse the content of the exchange and the accuracy and appropriacy of the interpreters' performance.

In both cases, it is important that the length of the video or video extract is suited to the objectives of the activity it is applied to, that its quality is good enough and that time is devoted to discussion of the video or on reflection on its content. The use of video may contribute to the development of almost all the competences from communicative and textual, with the study of specialist lexis in context, to the interpersonal with the interaction of the participants involved in the situation visualized, to the strategic competence and an analysis of the different types of interpreting skills used by the interpreter, for example.

Finally, videos are an incredibly versatile training tool: they can be paused, rewound, and viewed as many times as necessary, they appeal to learners with both visual and auditory learning styles and can be used both face-to-face and remotely, both in class and for autonomous study purposes.

3.3. *Sight translation (ST) exercises*

Despite the lack of a uniform definition of the concept of sight translation in applied linguistics studies (Krapivkina 2018), ST has been recognized as an important training method for interpreters (Ballardini 1998) even though, too often, it has only been used as a pedagogical tool for simultaneous and consecutive interpretation (Spilka 1966; Falbo 1995; Viaggio 1995) rather than for dialogue and therefore medical interpreting.

Nevertheless, in our experience, ST has proven to be a valid method to train medical interpreters as it helps trainees to shift from written to oral translation, to quickly find equivalents and/or synonyms in the foreign language, and to acquire speed, which is often key in medical settings where many situations in which interpreters find themselves are time-sensitive, such as, for example, in ER contexts. Moreover, ST is not just a pedagogical tool in medical interpreting but an actual everyday need: medical interpreters are often required to sight translate an old medical report to the doctor to enable them to make a diagnosis, an informed consent form to a patient before a procedure or the contents of a patient information leaflet of a drug.

Future medical interpreters should therefore practice sight translating medical texts in class, which can range from academic or newspaper articles on medical topics, if the goal is to improve terminology, speed and gather knowledge on a specific medical subfield and/or procedure, but also 'real life' texts such as doctor's reports, bureaucratic and informative documents, consent forms, patient information leaflets, etc., as these are good examples of actual texts they will be asked to sight translate in their future professional performance. Since this type of text is written to be read, not interpreted, and often contains very bureaucratic or technical language, practising sight translation in class will help learners to overcome such barriers and develop the skills to effectively convey their content to the patient or the doctor when on the job. Texts to be sight translated can also be included in roleplays to make things more complicated and to increase the feeling of a real situation, ideally in more advanced classes or for MA students. Sight translation is best performed in class under the guidance of a trainer, but in our experience, it was also successfully used as a training method in online courses, and students report that it was effectively employed as an autonomous study method both individually and in groups. Sight translation is probably key in the development of the communicative and textual, thematic and strategic competences.

3.4. Roleplays

Roleplays have been widely used, during the last thirty years, in community interpreters' training, as they promote participation, enhance engagement and allow students to experience different perspectives (Alden 1999; Schweickert and Heeren 1999; Kettula and Berghäll 2013) but most importantly because they 'reproduce the reality of services' (Niemants and Bernardi 2021) that cannot be experienced by observation or interpreting from a video source. The roleplays are intended to put the interpreting trainee in complex situations, which require rapid problem-solving and sometimes ethical challenges. There are different types of roleplays that can be used for training medical interpreters, all of which 'recreate' in class a real-life situation with three or more people who pretend to play a specific role (in our case, operator, patient and interpreter), by simulating what they would say in each situation based on indications provided by the trainer. It can be argued that they play a part in the development of all the competences and as such are an extremely versatile and useful training method.

If an entire script is provided to the operator and the patient, who are simply required to read/recite while the interpreter can practise rendering them in the other language, the roleplay is considered a 'scripted roleplay' of which an example is provided here in Figure 4.4. Scripted roleplays, which are the most commonly used, can be tailored to the level of the class, help students practise terminology, pronunciation, understanding and production and can be performed by the trainer (who will be usually performing the 'foreign person', whether patient or operator) and a student, although it is advisable, if possible, that two trainers are the primary interlocutors, each one of them in their native language, as we have noticed that students, when performing one of the roles tend to 'help' their fellow class mates by adapting language and pace, and are sometimes unable to act outside the script. Despite the many advantages of scripted roleplays, they are incredibly difficult and time-consuming for trainers to prepare, but most importantly they represent a 'close-ended' situation that leaves no space for improvisation, even though the 'actors', be they teacher or student, should be following the interpreter's rendition and not only what is written in the script. Also, no matter how hard we try to make the roleplay as authentic as possible, it is almost impossible to turn off the simulation frame completely, especially for students who have never actually experienced such situations (Niemants 2013).[3] In this respect, non-scripted roleplays, can offer more spontaneity as they only provide the operator (for example, doctor/patient) with general indications, or cue cards containing information about the character and about how the communicative situation should evolve, and participants are free to manage the conversation as they would do in real life. There are different levels of 'unscriptedness', and instructions

---

[3] This is why Niemants (2021) proposes combining RPs with the Conversational Analytic Roleplay Method (CARM), presenting records of authentic interactions with transcription, reflecting on problematic shifts and possible actions.

SCRIPTED ROLE-PLAY
Orthopaedics EN-EN

This role-play simulates a consultation in the ER orthopaedics department of a hospital in a tourist location (Rimini, Italy) between an English patient and the orthopaedists. The patient has already been triaged and x-ray has been taken and he has finally been called in to see a specialist. The consultation is carried out with help of the hospital's resident interpreter. The patient is one of the Liverpool football fans who have come to see the match against Sassuolo, some of whom have vandalized the city during the night after they lost 3-0.
In *italics* are some comments for trainers/trainees playing the role of the ORTHOPEDIST and/or the patient.
In green are instructions specific for the role-play readers and/or actors.

ORTHOPEDIST: So, you are Mr John Linconl, right? Born on 13.01.1955 right? (*To the interpreter while the interpreter is still speaking with an urgent and annoyed attitude*) Can you confirm it's him please?
PATIENT: **Yeah, it's me but it's spelled Lincoln, not Linconl.**
ORTHOPEDIST: (*grumbling*) Wonderful, those triage nurses wouldn't even be able to spell their own names, now it will take me ages to change the record.
Doctor fumbles and keeps writing on the computer ignoring both interpreter and patient
PATIENT: (*to the interpreter*) **What did he say?**
ORTHOPEDIST: So, here it says that you fell yesterday evening while amongst friends in a pub, and bumped your right arm and elbow, but you didn't come directly to the hospital and then this morning your shoulder hurt, and you went to see a doctor.
PATIENT: **Hem, well…yes, we came here for the UEFA Europa league match between Liverpool and Sassuolo, had a pint or two after the match, the floor was slippery in the pub, and I slipped and landed on my elbow and shoulder. The elbow is fine, just a bit bruised, but it's the shoulder that hurts the most. It didn't hurt yesterday so I thought a good night's sleep would do but then this morning I couldn't move it.**
ORTHOPEDIST: (*to the interpreter*) Well surely those pints helped to kill the pain, didn't they? He mustn't have been very sober, or he would have come earlier since he has a dislocated shoulder. (*To the patient*) On a scale from one to ten how would you evaluate your pain?
PATIENT: **It's throbbing… I'd say a 4.**
ORTHOPEDIST: A 4? This moron must still be drunk! (*To the interpreter*) Tell him that he's got a dislocated shoulder and a non-displaced upper arm bone fracture, next time stay at home my friend! Instead of vandalizing the city.
PATIENT: **What does that mean? Can you pop it in?**
ORTHOPEDIST: It means that the upper arm bone is forced out of the shoulder socket. Now we'll try the reduction manoeuvre if it works, or we'll have to go for surgery. And let's hope there is no lesion of the glenohumeral ligaments.
(*If the interpreter or the patient ask: glenohumeral ligaments are the ligaments in your shoulder joint*).
PATIENT: (*the patient has asked about both dislocation and displaced fracture. If the interpreter did not translate and explain the meaning of both*) **And what about my broken arm?**
ORTHOPEDIST: We'll try reduction for the fracture as well. Now, do you want a pain-killer for the arm?… I think it's even more painful than the reduction itself, but for the shoulder I'd suggest you take it.
PATIENT: **Oh no, don't worry I am a war veteran, 22nd Cheshire Regiment. I was wounded in Adraskan, Afghanistan, in 2011. I've still got a shrapnel fragment stuck into my leg. it's fine.**
ORTHOPEDIST: Are you sure?
PATIENT: **Hundred percent positive, sir.**

Figure 4.4. Scripted roleplay from the ReACTMe First Intensive Programme for Higher Education Learners on Medical Interpreting

Training Resources and Methodologies 145

can vary from quite detailed, or semi-scripted, as in Figure 4.5 to very few indications or 'cue cards'. This type of roleplay is easier and quicker to prepare for trainers, and much closer to 'a real interpreting situation', although more difficult to organize because they work best when a real healthcare operator is present.

SEMI-SCRIPTED ROLE-PLAY
ER EN-ES

This semi-scripted role-play recreates a triage acceptance at an hospital in Marbella, Spain, between a Spanish ER nurse at the triage and an English mother whose child is unconscious. We are at the triage in a very busy summer day.
For actors/readers: read carefully what you are required to do before hand, what you see there is just an indication to help you. The indication is the goal, what you are supposed to achieve, how you do you, how you ask questions, it is up to you.

PATIENT: You are a mother who gets in the ER with her child in her arms. You cry and ask for help in English.
NURSE: With the interpreter you try to figure out what's going on. Ask the relevant questions, what happened/how old is the child/are they from here....
PATIENT: You are from the UK on holiday. You were at the beach and the children's face got swollen up and he said he didn't feel well. The child is 5. But he does not speak well yet, so you only managed to see he was red and itchy, like mosquito bites. And he started to have breathing problems.
NURSE: Ask all the necessary questions on the children's medical history and the questions you would ask if you suspect an allergic reaction.
PATIENT: The child doesn't have a history of allergy, he is not asthmatic, but you are allergic to peanuts, almonds, shellfish. You are getting tense and anxious like you can't breathe. You tell the nurse everything the baby eat since early morning not to miss any important detail (tell a lot of food names).
NURSE: The mother is giving you uninfluential details and time is running and the child has been unconscious for two minutes. Saturation is bad. Tell the interpreter to cut the crap, you only want the last thing he ate. The case is serious, take out your phone and call doctor Alonso to come straightaway to the Emergency room where the respirator and all the stuff is.
PATIENT: When the interpreter interrupts you tell them the child had Nutella ice-cream.
NURSE: Ask the mother how long ago did the reaction start?
PATIENT: You are shocked, you cannot say. First you say one hour, then 20 minutes. In the end you decide for 20 minutes because you realise that he immediately passed out and you called an ambulance straightaway and came directly here.
OTHER DOCTOR: [*At this point while the interpreter is translating the nurse's words the interpreter's phone starts ringing. It's another doctor who is asking very abruptly to join him straight away in the Cardiology department for an urgent case*]
NURSE: You are annoyed at the interpreter. You want to reassure the mother, tell her you suspect sever anaphylaxis and that the thing you put in the child's veins is an IV drip with water and corticosteroids, explain what they are used for.

Figure 4.5. Semi or unscripted roleplay from the First Intensive Programme for Higher Education Learners

Finally, another type of roleplay that can be used in training medical interpreters is the multi-role roleplay, as it has been called by Garwood et al. (2023),[4] the colleague who devised this method, which is particularly suitable for multilingual classes. In this case the trainer prepares a script in a common language such as English, as in the case of the ReACTMe intensive programmes for higher education learners. The script is divided into three parts (A, B, C) and students are given their part of the script (either A, B or C) but they cannot see what happens in the other turns before practising and are left some time to prepare to interpret the shifts from the common language into their foreign language, to prepare terminology and imagine what other speakers will say. This is because the script is provided in English, and students will be asked to sight translate their turn in the relevant language. The class is then split in groups where one student plays the role of the healthcare provider (A), one plays the interpreter (B) and another the patient (C) as in a typical roleplay, with the trainer moving around and listening to the groups. After the activity, they meet all together with the trainer to discuss the difficulties encountered. The value of this type of roleplay lies in increasing participation, as every student is asked to interpret and therefore has more practice than they would with a normal roleplay. This type of roleplay can also be very useful when teaching multilingual classes, where trainees do not have the same language combinations, and it involves both roleplaying and sight translation. In our experience, roleplays of all types work better if performed under the guidance of a trainer in face-to-face contexts, although all three types were also used online in the ReACTMe First Intensive Programme for Higher Education Learners, which was held online, using break-out rooms for the multilingual activity.

The purpose of this type of learning activity, however it is implemented, is firstly to offer a 'real-life' situation for the future interpreter to engage and operate in, and secondly to improve vocabulary used in the two-language combination, note-taking skills, interaction management and problem-solving.

---

4   On the functioning of the Roleplay for multilingual classes, see Preziosi and Garwood (2017: 231–233).

3.5. Written texts

Texts are tools that can lead to the communicative acts targeted by the specific context of interpretation, that is, to a linguistic activity of a particular type, the final goal of which is the oral transposition, in another language, of a message addressed by speaker A to interlocutor B. The exercises proposed in the form of a written text are, in this respect, in line with the communicative learning teaching strategy, whereby students are asked to solve tasks that give them the ability to acquire new linguistic structures (especially specialized vocabulary in the medical field) in order to use it in situations of 'real communication' (Ellis 2003: 283). It might seem counterintuitive to use written texts to teach a profession that is mainly oral, but it is not if we consider that much of the information processed by our brains is visual, made up of images and text. In general, reading texts contributes to the development of certain automatisms, and specialized medical texts are no exception. Understanding the message, accumulating new information related to this specific topic, searching, finding and memorizing information and defining the field are just some of these automatisms. Written texts allow a better fixation of new vocabulary as, unlike spoken text, they can be returned to time and time again, providing a permanent record. Deducing the meaning of terms from context is simpler with written than with spoken texts owing to the permanence of the written word.

In addition, written text allows a quicker discovery of logical connectors, of the progression of the message, the evaluation and/or ranking of the degree of importance of the information which, in the interpretative process, are logical-intuitive and subject to the pressure of finding a functional solution in a very short time in the context, whereas in the case of processing written information they are the result of a deductive analysis.

To a certain extent, the written text presupposes reading skills first and foremost and reading will be, as Rouxel (2004: 18) defines it, 'sensitive to form, attentive to the functioning of the text'. In the case of medical texts, it will be sensitive to the informative dimension. In addition, the directive tone and nature of a medical leaflet or the persuasive nature of a recommendation for one treatment over another will help the student to find the right tone of interpretation for the message to be conveyed. The use of written texts can activate and develop logical skills as trainees establish relationships between various components of the text. In short, written texts can be employed for much-needed reflection about language and situations encountered in interpreting as a means of preparation for the rapid processing that interpreting requires. Written texts in medical interpreter training can therefore, to some extent, develop all the competences. As such they are extremely versatile, as they can be used successfully for online and asynchronous training, are easy to find, and can take the form of case studies, academic articles, informative texts from medical web pages, patient information leaflets, consent forms, doctors' notes, etc.

3.6. Terminology exercises

Terminology exercises are extremely useful in training medical interpreters as they build up vocabulary and acquaint students with both context and content, in addition to developing speed in finding equivalences. A trainee can go through a cardiology exercise, for example, and develop their knowledge about the different areas of the human heart in English, and can later do the same thing in Spanish, while reinforcing their knowledge of the content. What is important to stress here is that terminological exercises lead to a certain terminological competence, which is surely important but not sufficient in itself: with little or no understanding of the different branches of Medicine and their associated anatomy, diseases, diagnostic tests and treatments, the interpreter might know the corresponding term in another language but will struggle to perform in this field. For this reason, we believe, as Garwood and Tommassini (2023) point out in this volume, that it is better to present terminological exercises on a limited number of medical topics and subspecialities to provide future interpreters with some in-depth knowledge of some fields, rather than superficial knowledge in a wide range of topics. This selective approach to the study of terminology makes it easier for interpreters to prepare for assignments involving other illnesses or specialties as with in-depth study of specific areas they will acquire a methodology that can be applied to other fields. Terminological exercises are also useful to understand that sometimes there are not direct equivalents for cultural reasons to a specific term, or that there are different levels corresponding to different registers, and interpreters are thus called upon to reflect on the intercultural aspects of language mediation. Terminological exercises are suitable for both online and face-to-face training, although we have seen, in our ReACTMe experience, that they can very successfully be used for asynchronous learning, as students enjoy autonomy in the whole process of learning new terminology (Saienko and Chugai 2020) especially since recent studies (Kalay 2020) have shown that students are more stimulated to learn technical terminology in the digital environment. Terminology exercises are particularly relevant in the development of the communicative and textual and thematic competences.

4. Conclusions

In this short space, we have tried to outline the process and the results of research into resources and methods for the training of medical interpreters. We have presented how ReACTMe project members mapped existing resources and catalogued them, to later develop their own resources and reflect on the methods required to use those resources in medical interpreter training. In terms of resources, the ReACTMe project offers a mapping and categorization of resources which we believe will help teachers and trainers, as well as professional interpreters, to identify and meet specific training needs, and a collection of freely available original resources, specifically roleplays, terminological exercises, case studies and a multilingual glossary that can be employed immediately, or provide inspiration to trainers (for those with a different language combination) to create their own tasks.

As for methods, we have presented those methods that, we believe, contribute most to enhancing interpreters' professionality and skills, although the list is not extensive or exclusive and we would be happy to include more training methods to the list in the future. Among these methods, while all may be considered useful and effective, we felt, in our experience and following feedback from trainees and trainers in the training activities we organized, that terminological build-up and roleplays were particularly effective and appreciated, especially semi-scripted roleplays where real healthcare professionals were called in to participate. These were thought to provide an essential insight into the real world of interpreting.

As stated above, the project reviewed the literature available but also tapped into the experience of the members of the ReACTMe research team, both in their own universities and within this project's training experiences, to come up with a collection of resources. Such resources and methods might not be the best in absolute terms, but they proved to be effective in relative terms, that is in this time and place, and will surely need improvement as research into the profession and into training progresses. As our target was learners in higher education, both students of Medicine and interpreters, we adopted a broad approach but the target, if more specific, should always be taken into account by the trainer who will adapt the resources and methods to the class and to the type of learning required. Finally, we tried to offer resources that are free and available online and to include here reflections that considered both face-to-face and online training. The era of exclusively in-class learning ended with COVID-19 and although most classes are back to face-to-face mode, some parts of classes and of courses will be held asynchronously and online in the future. While this might be a challenge for trainers, it can also create new opportunities and facilitate a more personalized attention to our learners, which is surely a step in the right direction for education.

Bibliography

Alden, Dave.1999. 'Experience with scripted roleplay in environmental economics', *The Journal of Economic Education* 30(2), 127–132.
Angelelli, Claudia. 2019. *Healthcare Interpreting Explained.* London: Routledge.
Bain, Ken. 2004. *What the Best College Teachers Do.* Cambridge, MA: Harvard University Press.

Ballardini, Elio. 1998. 'La traduzione a vista nella formazione degli interpreti', *Intralinea* 1. <https://docenti.unimc.it/claudia.breviglieri/teaching/2015/15253/files/teoria-traduzione-a-vista>.

Bancroft, Marjory A., Katharine Allen, Carola E. Green, and Louis M. Feuerle. 2015. *Breaking Silence – Interpreting for Victims Services: A Training Manual*. Washington, DC: Ayuda.

Ellis, Rod. 2003. *Task Based Language Learning and Teaching*. Oxford: Oxford University Press.

Falbo, Caterina. 1995. 'Interprétation consecutive et exercises préparatoires', *The Interpreters' Newsletter* 6, 87–91.

Garwood, Christopher, Almudena Nevado Llopis, Ana Isabel Foulquié Rubio, Elena Tomassini, Alina Pelea, and Alina Andreica. 2023. 'Ethical dilemmas in medical interpreting – helping trainee interpreters decide', in Julian Bourne, M. Manuela Fernández Sánchez, Juncal Gutiérrez Artacho, Tatjana Portnova, E. Macarena Pradas Macías, and Enrique F. Quero Gervilla (eds) *Reflexiones sobre ética profesional de traductores e intérpretes y buenas prácticas*. Granada: Comares, 163–179

Herreid, Clyde. 2011.'Case study teaching', *New Directions for Teaching and Learning* 12, 31–40.

Kalay, Dilşah. 2020. 'Forming students' terminological competence in the Moodle-based E-Learning course', *Advanced Education* 16, 104–111.

Kettula, Kirsi, and Sami Berghäll. 2013. 'Drama-based role-play: A tool to supplement work-based learning in higher education', *Journal of Workplace Learning* 25(8), 556–575.

Krapivkina, Olga. 2018. 'Sight translation and its status in training of interpreters and translators', *Indonesian Journal of Applied Linguistics* 7(3), 695–704.

Nevado Llopis, Almudena, and Ana Isabel Foulquié Rubio. 2022. 'Recursos para la enseñanza-aprendizaje de la interpretación sanitaria: la base de datos de ReACTMe', in Monica Palmerini and Laura Mariottini (eds), *Estudios de Lingüística Hispánica: Teorías, datos, contextos y aplicaciones*. Madrid: Dykinson, 1671–1698.

Niemants, Natacha. 2013. 'From role-playing to role-taking: Interpreter role(s) in healthcare', in Christina Schäffner, Krzysztof Kredens, and Yvonne Fowler (eds), *Interpreting in a Changing Landscape: Selected Papers from Critical Link 6*. Amsterdam: John Benjamins, 305–319.

Niemants, Natacha. 2021. 'Teoria e prassi dell'interpretazione dialogica', in Mariachiara Russo (ed,), *Interpretare da e verso l'italiano: proposte didattiche e innovazione*. Bologna: Bononia University Press, 41–60.

Niemants, Natacha, and Eleonora Bernardi. 2021. 'Interpretare per i servizi sociosanitari', in Mariachiara Russo (ed.), *Interpretare da e verso l'italiano: proposte didattiche e innovazione*. Bologna: Bononia University Press, 395–414.
PACTE, Grupo. 2001. 'La competencia traductora y su adquisición', *Quaderns. Revista de Traducció* 6, 39–45.
Pöchhacker, Franz. 2004. *Introducing Interpreting Studies*. London: Routledge.
Preziosi, Ira, and Christopher Garwood. 2017. 'Training legal interpreters in an imperfect world', in Letizia Cirillo and Natacha Niemants (eds), *Teaching Dialogue Interpreting: Research-Based Proposals for Higher Education*. Amsterdam: John Benjamins, 217–238.
Rouxel, Annie. 2004. 'Qu'entend-on par lecture littéraire', in Catherine Tauveron (ed.), *La Lecture et la culture littéraires au cycle des approfondissements*. CRDP de Versailles: Canopé.
Rybarczyk, Brian. 2017. 'A case-based approach increases student learning outcomes and comprehension of cellular respiration concepts', *Methods* 35, 181–186.
Saienko, Nataliia, and Oksana Chugai. 2020. 'Quarantine: Teaching English from home with Google Classroom, Classtime and Quizlet', *Revista Romaneasca Pentru Educatie Multidimensionala* 12(1), 151–156.
Sawyer, David. 2004. *Fundamental Aspects of Interpreter Education: Curriculum and Assessment*. Amsterdam: John Benjamins.
Schweickert, Eileen, and Allison Heeren. 1999. 'Scripted roleplay: A technique for teaching sexual history taking', *The Journal of the American Osteopathic Association* 99(5), 275–276. <https://doi.org/10.7556/jaoa.1999.99.5.275>.
Spilka, Irène. 1966. 'La traduction à vue instrument de formation', *Meta* 11(2), 43–45.
Viaggio, Sergio. 1995. 'The praise of sight translation (and squeezing the last drop thereout of)', *The Interpreters' Newsletter* 4, 45–58.

CHRISTOPHER GARWOOD

5 Key Elements to Be Considered When Designing a Course for Medical Interpreters

As explained in the previous chapters, interpreting in healthcare settings presents a number of very specific challenges, in addition to the usual challenges faced in any kind of dialogue interpreting. Any course aimed at training medical interpreters must clearly identify these challenges for students to be able to develop the competences they require to perform adequately as interpreters in healthcare settings and include lessons, materials and activities that promote the development of these competences.[1]

    These guidelines are based on the combined didactic and practical interpreting experience of all the members of the ReACTMe project, a review of the literature, an analysis of existing courses and the testing of lessons, materials and activities during three intensive five-day pilot training activities organized as part of the ReACTMe project.[2] The guidelines are intended to help higher education institutions (HEIs) and trainers design

1   The core competences identified in the field of MI are: interpreting competence, interpersonal communication skills, intercultural competence, linguistic competence, ethical competence, medical competence, contextual/thematic competence and self-care competence. The learning outcomes associated with each competence can be found in Chapter 6 of this volume, describing the Joint Blended Module on Medical Interpreting. It should be noted that, in both the literature and practice, the name given to these competences may sometimes vary (Training Resources Compilation on the ReACTMe Learning Platform, <http://reactme.net/learning-platform/training-resources-compilation>), but the associated knowledge, skills and attitudes remain the same.

2   Short-Term Staff Training Event C1 (Cluj – online), a training for trainers in which trainers also played the part of students to test various ideas and materials; First Intensive Programme for Higher Education Learners C2 (Rome – online),

and implement Medical Interpreting (MI) courses, offering ideas as regards not only the types of lessons, materials and activities we believe to be most effective in such a course,[3] but also as regards course structure, organization, modality and curriculum.

After highlighting non-didactic factors that may sometimes be overlooked, we outline the main ideas and principles of what we believe to be an efficient and effective structure and organization for an MI course. We then provide a general description of materials and activities that we believe to be most useful in this kind of course. Actual examples regarding course structure, organization, materials and activities will be provided by referring to the Joint Blended Extracurricular Module on Medical Interpreting, a stand-alone course in MI developed as one of the intellectual outputs of the ReACTMe project, which offers a practical example of an MI course, including sample lessons, materials and activities.

1. Before getting started

Before starting to design a course in MI, however, there are a number of external factors that can have a major impact on course design, above all, its length, which, in turn, affects the level that can be achieved in terms of the various competences. The first question to ask is whether there is a need for such a course. From the national surveys carried out as part of the ReACTMe project, the answer in the three project countries is undoubtedly yes, but for what languages? The answer to that question varies both geographically and over time. It is also necessary to find out

---

involving students from the six participating universities; and Second Intensive Programme for Higher Education Learners C3 (Murcia – face-to-face), once more involving students from the six participating universities.

3   This will also provide students wanting to learn how to become medical interpreters with useful guidance as to what and how they should be studying. These guidelines are not intended, however, as a 'Teach Yourself How to Become a Medical Interpreter' textbook.

how much medical interpreters are paid, as this will greatly determine how much people are willing to invest in such a course in terms of both time and money, which has a strong bearing on the cost and length of the course.

After deciding on the length and cost of a course, it is then necessary to calculate how many students need to enrol for the course to be financially sustainable, as it is extremely unlikely, nowadays, that a HEI would authorize a course that is not financially sustainable. Is this number of students possible with just one foreign language (L2) or will it be necessary to have a multilingual course with various L2s? Will there be enough people wanting to follow an MI course in just one L2 and is there enough work for medical interpreters with that L2?[4] Will the course be aimed exclusively at students who have already received formal interpreter training? If not, will those without formal training be expected to have practical interpreting experience? Will students without training be given additional support (an extra cost) at the beginning of the course? These are all questions that must be answered before even starting to design a course.

Another important factor to consider is the resources available at your HEI. These include, above all, human resources (such as trainers with MI experience and the availability of healthcare professionals willing to be involved in the course), institutional resources (including the availability of classrooms, especially at weekends, as required in our case) and technical resources, of particular importance for a course adopting a blended-learning approach (our case), involving both asynchronous learning (using materials and activities made available via an online learning platform) and synchronous learning in both face-to-face and online modalities. The availability or lack of availability of such resources at your HEI will also affect the design and cost of the course.

All these various factors must be taken into consideration before starting to design an MI course since a course that may be perfect on paper, with excellent learning outcomes, may be totally unrealistic in terms of cost

---

4   A multilingual MI course is rather more difficult to organize and the level that can be attained is generally slightly lower than in a course with just one L2, though in our personal experience students often find multilingual courses more stimulating.

and length in relation to the demand for such a course and the job opportunities that exist. The starting point when designing an MI course must, therefore, be some form of business plan in order to have a more realistic idea of the kind of course that can be created.

2. Course structure and organization

Once you have a clearer idea of the intended participants of the course, its length and the languages involved, the next aspect to focus on is the structure and organization of the course. These guidelines are intended to help in the design of MI courses that, in addition to successfully training medical interpreters to a suitable level, are also cost-effective by making the best possible use of the time students spend both together with their trainers and when working on their own.

This is one of the reasons why we chose a blended-learning approach for our model course, the Joint Blended Extracurricular Module on Medical Interpreting, where lectures, materials and activities are provided via an online platform for asynchronous learning. There are other important reasons, however. First and foremost, we believe that any MI course should be truly student-centred, giving students far greater responsibility in how and what they learn, especially in the case of a stand-alone module such as this. A key feature of a student-centred approach is the use of flipped learning, where students are given material to prepare on specific topics that will then be the subject of the lessons with their trainers in the classroom, thereby prioritizing active learning when trainers are present. Working asynchronously, students also have far greater flexibility as they can choose not only when is most suitable for them to engage in this preparatory work, but also how they study the material. What is essential, here, is to select materials that can be studied equally well or even better asynchronously.

In the blended module we propose, some of the lessons with the trainers are also delivered online as, while, in our collective experience, there is a general preference for face-to-face lessons among both trainers and students, the recent imposed switch to online learning/teaching during the COVID-19 pandemic has provided both trainers and students with considerable experience in the online modality and shown that excellent results can be achieved in interpreting courses in this modality as well.[5] The asynchronous learning and the delivery of some of the lessons online result in important savings in both time and money – no transport costs, no need to hire classrooms, no time wasted travelling, etc. – making the course less costly and more student-friendly.

As regards the structure of the course, as in the case of the Joint Blended Extracurricular Module on Medical Interpreting, intended as a stand-alone module to be held at weekends so that people who work can also attend, we propose a cyclical structure in order to make the best possible use of the blended approach, with a division into Weeks A, B and C. After a one-day introductory session, there is a Week A, which consists in online asynchronous learning, when students independently study material provided via an online platform in preparation for the lessons and activities of Weeks B and C, with each cycle focusing primarily on one specific branch of Medicine. In Week B, the lessons are face-to-face (Friday afternoons and all day on Saturday) and mainly involve interpreting practice and discussion, while in Week C the lessons and activities are held online, with the students working together in groups on their own (Friday afternoons) and then together with their trainers (Saturday mornings) to reinforce the work done during Weeks A and B. In our 60-hour module,[6] this cyclical structure is repeated four times, but this number can, obviously, be reduced or increased as required.

---

[5] This was also the opinion of the trainers as regards the two ReACTMe pilot training activities for higher education learners, the first of which (C2 Rome) was held online, while the second (C3 Murcia) was face-to-face. The students' course evaluations were also extremely positive in both cases.

[6] The 60 hours refer to the contact hours with trainers for synchronous work, while the total workload of the module, including autonomous work, is 150–180 hours (6 ECTS). The majority of the ReACTMe partners felt that this was the most likely length of the course at their institutions, but both shorter and longer courses were considered.

In our case, the four major topics chosen for the four cycles are Cardiology, Orthopaedics, Maternity Care and Emergency Care. Maternity Care and Emergency Care would seem to be essential topics in any MI course, while Orthopaedics and Cardiology, clearly important topics in their own right, are also both very useful in relation to Emergency Care. If there are any prevalent illnesses among the local foreign-speaking population, they would be a natural topic to study. The availability of someone with expertise in a specific topic can be a good reason for selecting that topic as they are also able to provide valuable insights.[7] The most important thing, however, is to focus on just a few topics, studying in depth the relevant anatomy and physiology, associated diseases and symptoms, the most common relevant diagnostic tests and the treatment provided. In this way, students acquire a good medical competence in addition to terminological competence, as opposed to a very superficial knowledge when a wide range of topics are studied. At best, this results in a certain terminological competence, but with little or no understanding of the different branches of Medicine and their associated anatomy, diseases, diagnostic tests and treatment. The in-depth medical knowledge acquired focusing on just a few topics also makes it easier for interpreters to prepare for assignments involving other illnesses as they also acquire a methodology.

In addition to the specific branches of Medicine, these cycles of lessons also include topics related to other competences, such as knowledge of how the national health system works, who has access to the system, the workplace environment, ethical issues, cultural issues, self-care, etc. These other topics should be included where most appropriate in the course programme and must then be present in the interpreting activities the students engage in during that cycle.

---

7   In fact, Cardiology was also chosen because of the specific expertise of one of the members of the ReACTMe team, with a wealth of knowledge and materials on the topic.

3. Teaching/learning materials

The choice of the materials used in an MI course is, clearly, of paramount importance and will have a decisive role in the outcome of the course. It is essential, therefore, for course and lesson designers to have a very clear idea of what they are trying to achieve with the materials they are proposing. They must also ensure that there is sufficient connection between the materials given to the students to prepare in Week A and the materials used for the activities, above all for interpreting practice, in Weeks B and C.

3.1. Background material (Week A)

There is a vast amount of materials already available on whatever branches of Medicine are chosen as the major topics for in-depth study and these can often be used exactly as they are or adapted to suit the specific needs of trainers. As students study the topic on their own, a key concept with regard to the background materials is 'graduality', which means that the first materials they are given to study on the major topic should be of a more generalist nature. Once they have acquired a basic knowledge, the next materials should be more technical, so they also acquire the necessary terminology. It is important, however, not to overload students by giving them too many materials to study. In our 6 ECTS module, students are not expected to do more than 8–10 hours study during Week A. Given that students are working on their own, variety is also advisable with regard to the materials they are asked to study. Written texts are simpler to acquire knowledge of a new subject, after which students can also be given videos to watch and study, especially as they can help them with the pronunciation of more technical terms. It is advisable to provide exercises to enable students to self-assess how much they have managed to learn on the topic. In this respect, there are numerous exercises on the ReACTMe Learning Platform that can be used for this purpose (<http://reactme.net/learning-platform>).

3.2. *Sight translation*

Sight translation is a necessary skill for interpreters working in healthcare settings as they are often called upon to orally translate written documents, such as consent forms patients must sign before undergoing certain medical examinations or surgery (L1 into L2) or patients' records (L2 into L1). The various forms can be given as materials to be studied in Week A or worked on during specific lessons, after which they should be included in role plays in situations where these documents would need to be orally translated.

Sight translation can also be practised using other types of materials, including background materials, especially as a preparatory activity for students who have had no prior interpreter training.

3.3. *Monolingual videos*

We advise the use of monolingual training videos produced for students of Medicine or Nursing to show them how to interact with patients in different kinds of situations for initial interpreting practice on a topic. Specifically developed by medical practitioners, these videos in L1 usually offer realistic depictions of doctor-patient or nurse-patient encounters. In addition to providing excellent interpreting practice from L1 to L2, they also enable students to gain insights into various types of interactions between doctor/nurse and patient in a monolingual setting. After using the videos for interpreting practice, the videos should then be studied to analyse these interactions in terms of the language used, the various strategies employed by doctors/nurses to elicit information, the order in which questions are asked to obtain the information, etc. Trainers need to ensure that all these different aspects emerge when discussing these encounters with their students as students must become familiar with the interactions between doctor/nurse and patient in a monolingual situation in order to know what should ideally be happening when they interpret for a foreign-speaking patient.

While a vast selection of such teaching videos is available in English, it is now much easier to find them in many other languages as well. Alternatively, it is not too difficult or costly to produce videos of this kind in-house (under the guidance of healthcare practitioners).

3.4. Roleplays

After monolingual videos, roleplays[8] become the main activity for interpreting practice. In order to be effective teaching/learning tools, however, roleplays must be carefully designed in line with the competences that trainers want their students to develop through them. If trainers want to focus on, for example, ethical or cultural issues, then they must be appropriately scripted into the dialogues of the medical encounters that students will be asked to interpret. Roleplays must also be realistic if they are to be taken seriously by students, so it is advisable for trainers without the necessary personal experience to get healthcare professionals to check the scripts. Roleplays are also widely used in the training of doctors and nurses, so trainers can easily find every kind of roleplay, which can then be adapted by trainers to suit their specific needs.

There are three main types of roleplays: scripted roleplays, unscripted roleplays and multi-role roleplays. In the case of the ReACTMe module (and the two pilot training activities – C2 and C3), bilingual scripted roleplays are activities to be performed in front of the class, with trainers playing the parts of both the healthcare professional and the patient, and one or more students playing the part of the interpreter. Trainers, through their experience and having either designed or, at least, carefully studied the roleplays, are not only able to play the parts more realistically, but also know how to adapt the roleplays and keep them on track when interpreters diverge from the script. Performed in front of the class, these roleplays enable trainers to highlight what student interpreters manage to do both

---

8 There are several bilingual scripted roleplays (combining English, Spanish, Italian and Romanian) on the ReACTMe Learning Platform that can be downloaded and used for interpreting practice.

successfully and less successfully, providing feedback the entire class can learn from. In this way, students have a much clearer idea of what they should be doing and not doing when they practise without the supervision of their trainers.

Unscripted roleplays, which require the involvement of people with professional experience of working in the settings and situations chosen for the roleplay, are more spontaneous and offer greater variety, but there is, obviously, less control over the content. That is also why this type of roleplay is best offered later on in a course, after students have acquired a reasonable level of competence in MI.

Multi-role roleplays are a form of scripted roleplay, but with some important differences. The main idea of these roleplays is to give all the students an opportunity not only to practise their interpreting, but also to play the role of both the healthcare professional and the patient. Seeing the roleplay from these different perspectives, they gain a better understanding of the interactions in which they are involved. The students are first divided into groups of three and given script A (healthcare professional-interpreter-patient), script B (patient-healthcare professional-interpreter) or script C (interpreter-patient-healthcare professional). They are then given around thirty minutes to prepare their parts together with the other students who have their same script (A, B or C), also because the script is in the 'wrong' language (the part of the healthcare professional is in L_2, but they have to play the part in L_1, and vice versa for the patient).[9] Students are instructed

9   In the case of multilingual courses, where there are several different L_2s, the multi-role roleplay is an essential form of interpreting practice as bilingual roleplays require the translation of one part of the script into all the different L_2s, which is extremely costly. It functions slightly differently, however. To take advantage of the presence of the different L_2s, rather than having groups in which everyone has the same L_2, the groups of three comprise two students with the same L_2 and one student with a different L_2, with the latter playing the part of the healthcare professional (all the scripts are in L_1, so they just have to study the script). The two students with the same L_2 play, alternately, the part of the patient (they have to prepare the script in L_2) and that of the interpreter. This makes the roleplay more realistic as the student playing the part of the healthcare professional is totally dependent on the interpreter when it comes to communicating with the patient, making it essential for the student to study the part carefully to be able to react and

to use the thirty minutes not only to resolve any translation problems, but also to fully understand the parts they are playing, so they can improvise when necessary. They are also told to discuss what they think will happen in the part when they are the interpreter on the basis of the two parts they have been preparing. Improvisation by the doctor and patient in these roleplays is often rendered necessary by the script itself,[10] in addition to the influence the interpretation may have on the interaction.

After this preparation, students perform the roleplay in their groups of three, without the constant supervision of their trainers, who pass from one group to another, merely observing. At the end of the roleplay, students give their feedback on the interpreting performances in their individual groups, before a general discussion among the whole class as regards the problems encountered, possible solutions and any other aspects of interest, with trainers highlighting important elements that emerge and offering translation and strategic solutions.

This form of roleplay is truly student-centred and has proved to be very empowering for students, enabling them to practise similar-to-real-life situations without the fear of failure or of being judged in front of their peers, while the preparation stage helps to create a more collaborative environment. The need for students to be able to assess their peers also requires students to assume greater responsibility. And, of particular importance, everyone gets to practise.

For this kind of activity to be truly effective, however, students need to have a clear idea of what they should be doing when interpreting, of the strategies they should be using when facing a problem, and of the things they should be avoiding. The scripted roleplays in front of the class followed by discussion are essential for this to be possible. If there is no objection on the part of students, it is a good idea to video/audio record

---

bring the script back on track whenever it deviates. Students take turns at playing this part as there is no interpreting practice for them, but they usually find seeing the roleplay from this viewpoint extremely educational.

10 For example, the patient is scripted to say something directly to the interpreter, who will react in some way, while the healthcare professional is instructed in the script to ask what is going on.

the roleplays to analyse the performance of the interpreters (and the role players) in even greater detail.

Where possible, the materials used for interpreting practice (videos, roleplays, consent forms, etc.) should be reused for other purposes, such as the analysis and discussion of ethical and cultural issues, interpersonal communication, power asymmetry and empathy, a useful way of doing the most with all the materials prepared for the training.

ELENA TOMASSINI

6 A Model Joint Blended-Learning Module for Medical Interpreters[1]

1. Programme

Here, below, is the programme of the Joint Blended Extracurricular Module on Medical Interpreting, including the types of materials and activities proposed, with links to actual materials for activities that will be described in more detail in Section 3.

2. Competences and learning outcomes

As for the competences to be developed by the students participating in this module, as well as the learning outcomes associated to these competences, they are described in the following table.

---

1 An adapted version of this model was successfully implemented by the University of Bologna's Department of Interpretation and Translation in 2023 as a 72-hour professional development course and was well received by the participants. It is expected to be implemented by the other partner universities in the near future, with the exemption of Iuliu Hațieganu University of Medicine and Pharmacy.

Table 6.1. Programme of the Joint Blended Extracurricular Module

	JOINT BLENDED EXTRACURRICULAR MODULE ON MEDICAL INTERPRETING
	Weeks A: Students work autonomously at home using asynchronous materials provided by the trainers via the online learning platform.
	Weeks B: Classes face-to-face with trainers.
	Weeks C: Students work online in groups with their peers (Friday) and with their trainers (Saturday).
	There will also be a forum on the learning platform where students can meet, discuss and find solutions to any problems they may have.
	(6 ECTS = 60 contact hours and 150/180 total hours work)
WEEK 1 (B)	
Saturday 105 min	*Introduction to the course* Medical interpreting (MI) Course Structure Teaching Methods
Coffee break (15 min)	
120 min	Introduction to medical knowledge: Basic anatomy and physiology; common diseases, disorders and injuries and their treatment; the main diagnostic techniques, for example, blood tests, urine tests, imaging techniques (MRI, ultrasound, x-ray, PET, etc.). Discussion.
Lunch break (60 min)	
120 min	Introduction to medical terminology Meaning of frequently used prefixes and suffixes and common Latin and Greek roots, as well as common collocations. Practice and discussion.

Table 6.1. Continued

WEEK 2 (A) CARDIOLOGY	Cardiology
	Easy-to-understand text on the anatomy and physiology of the heart, common heart illnesses and conditions (types, causes and symptoms), diagnostic tests and treatments. <www.webmd.com/heart-disease/heart-disease-types-causes-symptoms> Similar text using a more technical language. <www.mayoclinic.org/diseases-conditions/heart-disease/symptoms-causes/syc-20353118> Video explaining the specific medical terminology of cardiology through the meanings of prefixes, suffixes and Latin and Greek root terms (reinforcing the knowledge acquired in Week 1). <https://youtu.be/nWRDYkB9IHU> Exercises to test and consolidate knowledge of cardiology (using those developed for the ReACTMe Learning Platform). National healthcare legislation and regulations <www.gov.uk/guidance/nhs-entitlements-migrant-health-guide> Access to the healthcare system for foreign citizens (e.g. appointments and referral procedures, payments, exemptions, etc.). Students asked to identify differences from healthcare systems of L2 countries. For trainees with a medical background, material explaining the various competences that must be developed for interpreting together with exercises to develop these competences to be uploaded onto the learning platform.

(continued)

Table 6.1. Continued

WEEK 3 (B) CARDIOLOGY	
Friday 180 min	History taking Introduction to how a patient's clinical history is taken using the SOCRATES method. Discussion. Monolingual video of a nurse taking the clinical history of a diabetic patient. After interpreting the video into L2, students watch the video again to observe the SOCRATES method in action and begin to understand the principles behind medical communication. Practice and discussion. <https://youtu.be/gsjKcQUsQY8> [Short break] A second monolingual video, this time of a doctor speaking to a patient with chest pains, for further interpreting practice into L2 and then to observe other ways in which doctors elicit information. Practice and discussion. <https://youtu.be/9om2tedf900>
Saturday 120 min	Scripted bilingual roleplay with trainers playing both parts. Practice and discussion.
Coffee break (15 min)	
75 min	Ethics: Ethical dilemmas questionnaire (1). Introduction to codes of ethics with examples of well-known codes of ethics. The deontological vs teleological approach to ethical dilemmas. Discussion.
30 min	Introduction to different types of roleplays – scripted roleplays, multi-role roleplays and unscripted roleplays.
Lunch break (60 min)	
180 min	Multi-role roleplay dealing with a case of angina. Practice and discussion. [Short break] Explanation of how trainees will work together in the activities to be done together online in Week C.

Table 6.1. Continued

WEEK 4 (C) CARDIOLOGY	
Friday 180 min	Monolingual video of doctor visiting a patient with a cardiological complaint using the SOCRATES method. Students work in groups of 3, with the video divided into three parts, one of which they have been assigned to prepare beforehand, so they know when to pause the video and can give the necessary feedback, also terminological, when discussing interpreter performance. Practice and discussion. <https://youtu.be/ECs9O5zl6XQ> [Short break] History taking: Interpreting practice in groups of three followed by peer discussion.
Saturday 105 min	Interpreting of monolingual video of a cardiological examination, also providing a further example of medical communication. The doctor takes the history of a patient suffering from chest pain, asking the patient about his family's medical history, his smoking and alcohol habits, treatment he is receiving, before informing him about what is going to happen. Practice and discussion. <https://youtu.be/8wdrG1Ct8og>
Coffee break (15 min)	
90 min	Multi-role roleplay on cardiac examination in groups of three. Practice and discussion.

(continued)

Table 6.1. Continued

WEEK 5 (A) ORTHOPAEDICS	Orthopaedics Easy-to-understand texts on the musculoskeletal system, common injuries, diseases and congenital disorders (types, causes and symptoms), diagnostic tests and treatment (including arthroscopy and arthroplasty). <https://my.clevelandclinic.org/health/body/12254-musculoskeletal-system-normal-structure--function> Video on new orthopedic imaging technologies and modalities. <https://youtu.be/zkcCPMzZDF0> For trainees with a medical background, further exercises to develop their interpreting competence on the learning platform.
WEEK 6 (B) ORTHOPAEDICS	
Friday 120 min	Interpreting of monolingual video of doctor visiting patient. Practice and discussion. [Short break]
60 min	Presentation on the importance of workplace knowledge, for example, the location of the different departments, in a hospital and the identification of hospital staff and their different roles (uniforms). Discussion.
Saturday 120 min	Interpreting of scripted bilingual roleplay involving an orthopaedic visit with trainers playing both parts performed in front of the class. Practice and discussion.
Coffee break (15 min)	
105 min	Presentation on intercultural issues, including topics such as pain and physical contact (psychologically invasive). Discussion.
Lunch break (60 min)	
120 min	Multi-role roleplay on orthopaedics in groups of three. Practice and discussion. [Short break]
60 min	The roles of interpreters in MI. Discussion.

Table 6.1. Continued

WEEK 7 (C) ORTHOPAEDICS	
Friday 90 min	Interpreting of monolingual video of doctor carrying out an orthopaedic examination. Students work in groups of 3, with the video divided into three parts, one of which they have been assigned to prepare beforehand. Practice and discussion. [Short break]
90 min	Monolingual videos on imaging. Practice and discussion. [Short break]
Saturday 90 min	Scripted bilingual roleplay on orthopaedics with trainers playing both parts. Practice and discussion.
Coffee break (15 min)	
105 min	Multi-role roleplay on orthopaedics in groups of three. Practice and discussion.
WEEK 8 (A) MATERNITY CARE	Maternity Care Texts describing different stages of maternity care (antenatal, delivery and postnatal) – procedures, complications, common diseases and disorders, diagnostic tests and treatment. (Inter)cultural issues in maternity care.
WEEK 9 (B) MATERNITY CARE	
Friday 120 min	Interpreting of monolingual video of doctor visiting pregnant woman. Practice and discussion. [Short break]
60 min	Presentation on (inter)cultural issues in the field of maternity care. Discussion.
Saturday 105 min	Patient's history taking on maternity care. Practice and discussion.

(*continued*)

Table 6.1. Continued

Coffee break (15 min)	
120 min	Scripted bilingual roleplay on maternity care with trainers playing both parts – practice and discussion.
Lunch break (60 min)	
90 min	Multi-role roleplay on maternity care in groups of 3 – practice and discussion.
60 min	(Inter)cultural issues and ethical dilemmas in maternity care. Discussion.
WEEK 10 (C) MATERNITY CARE	
Friday 120 min	Patient's history taking. Practice and discussion. [Short break]
120 min	Interpreting of monolingual video of doctor visiting pregnant patient in groups of three. Practice and discussion.
Saturday 90 min	Scripted bilingual roleplay on maternity care with trainers playing both parts. Practice and discussion.
Coffee break (15 min)	
105 min	Multi-role roleplay on self-care in groups of three. Practice and discussion.
WEEK 11 (A) EMERGENCY CARE	No specific material to be studied asynchronously.
WEEK 12 (B) EMERGENCY CARE	
Friday 120 min	Presentation on working in Emergency Care. Discussion. Scripted bilingual roleplay on emergency care with trainers playing both parts – practice and discussion. [Short break]

Table 6.1. Continued

60 min	Presentation on stress and vicarious trauma – self-care (coping strategies, including use of the third person). Discussion.
Saturday 105 min	Interpreting monolingual video of doctor examining a patient using the Four Frames Approach. Practice and discussion. <https://youtu.be/vlfdybUCzFw>
Coffee break (15 min)	
120 min	Monolingual video explaining the SPIKES approach to breaking bad news. Discussion. <www.youtube.com/watch?v=cg2v97-9z9s> Interpreting monolingual video of doctor breaking bad news using the SPIKES approach. Practice and discussion. <www.youtube.com/watch?v=_uOS7hfKkVI>
Lunch break (60 min)	
120 min	Multi-role roleplay on SPIKES model in groups of three. Practice and discussion. [Short break]
60 min	Relaxation techniques.
WEEK 13 (C) EMERGENCY CARE	
Saturday 120 min	Multi-role roleplay on emergency care in groups of three. Practice and discussion.
Coffee break (15 min)	
75 min	Ethical dilemmas questionnaire (2), course questionnaire, discussion.
Lunch	All together – students and trainers

Source: ReACTMe researchers

Table 6.2. Competences to be developed by the students attending the module and their associated learning outcomes

Required Competences	Learning Outcomes At the end of the course, students will be able to…
Interpreting Skills	… provide an appropriate interpreting service in a wide range of healthcare situations.
Medical Competence	… have a basic knowledge of Medicine: anatomy, human body systems, the most prevalent illnesses and injuries, and the main diagnostic tests and procedures.
Ethical Competence	… be familiar with the concepts contained in the most important professional codes of ethics for medical interpreters to help them behave in a professional manner at all times, never allowing their opinions or values to interfere with the interpreting interaction.
Information-Mining Competence	… carry out documentary and terminological research on the internet or using any other medium.
Intercultural Competence	… understand cross-cultural differences and/or barriers to prevent or resolve possible conflicts, considering a patient's cultural beliefs in relation to diet, illness and disease, etc.
Interpersonal Communication Competence	… clearly inform healthcare providers and patients of the interpreter's role before starting interpreting; suggest the best seating arrangements; ask all parties to use the first person and to avoid engaging in any kind of private conversation with the interpreter; and manage turn-taking.
Linguistic Competence	… master their working languages (and their different registers), all the most frequent terms and expressions used in healthcare encounters, including collocations, the terminology regarding body systems and the main diseases and diagnostic tests; and understand the prefixes and suffixes used in medical terminology, as well as the most frequent abbreviations.

Table 6.2. Continued

Required Competences	Learning Outcomes At the end of the course, students will be able to…
Self-Care Competence	… understand and recognize the consequences deriving from working in highly emotional situations; know their limitations and take care of their mental and physical well-being; use coping strategies to tackle highly emotional situations to reduce stress and psychological difficulties (such as the use of the third person instead of the first person or requesting a briefing session when bad news have to be delivered); and be familiar with stress-relieving techniques.
Thematic/ Contextual Competence	… know how their national and regional healthcare systems work, including relevant procedures, such as appointment and referral systems; know the various healthcare professionals' roles; know how healthcare facilities, such as a hospital (personnel, wards, outpatient clinics, etc.), admission procedures, triage and medical records are organized.

Source: ReACTMe researchers

3. Course content and examples of course materials

The course materials described here can either be accessed via the link or are available on the ReACTMe Learning Platform (e.g. Cardiology exercises).

3.1. Week 1

3.1.1. Introduction to interpreting techniques and skills

Outline: A presentation should be prepared to present the specificities of medical interpreting, the skills and techniques required, and the particular difficulties of this context, such as the emotional burden.

Competences to be acquired: Interpreting, medical, ethical, intercultural, interpersonal, linguistic and self-care competence. Students will immediately understand that all these competences are interrelated.

3.1.2. Introduction to medical knowledge for medical interpreters

A presentation should be prepared to provide and introduction to medical knowledge for medical interpreters.

Outline: This presentation will introduce the medical knowledge essential for medical interpreters, starting with a brief introduction to basic anatomy and physiology; common diseases, disorders and injuries, and their treatment; and the main diagnostic techniques, such as blood tests, urine tests and imaging techniques (MRI, ultrasound, x-ray, PET, etc.).

Competences to be acquired: Medical, linguistic and thematic/contextual competence.

3.1.3. Introduction to medical terminology

A presentation should be prepared to explain the meaning of frequently used prefixes and suffixes and common Latin and Greek roots.

Outline: This presentation will analyse combined forms present in medical terminology and provide a few simple exercises to highlight how it is possible in this way to decipher the meaning of medical terms.

Competences to be acquired: Linguistic, medical and interpreting competence.

3.2. Week 2 (Cardiology – A)

3.2.1. Introductory texts

<www.webmd.com/heart-disease/heart-disease-types-causes-symptoms>

Outline: Easy-to-understand text on the anatomy and physiology of the heart, common heart illnesses and conditions (types, causes and symptoms), diagnostic tests and treatments.

Competences to be acquired: Linguistic, medical and thematic/contextual competence.

<www.mayoclinic.org/diseases-conditions/heart-disease/symptoms-causes/syc-20353118>

Outline: Text using a more technical language to describe the most common heart diseases, including their symptoms, causes, risk factors. There are also videos, illustrations and a link to the Diagnosis and Treatment Section.

Competences to be acquired: Medical and linguistic competence.

<https://youtu.be/nWRDYkB9IHU>

Outline: Video presenting medical terms relating to the cardiovascular system, explaining prefixes, suffixes and root terms, developing the knowledge acquired during the introductory lesson on medical terminology.

Competences to be acquired: Linguistic, medical and interpreting competence.

3.2.2. Introduction to the National Health System

<www.gov.uk/guidance/nhs-entitlements-migrant-health-guide>

Outline: Text explaining how foreign citizens can access the National Health Service (NHS) in the United Kingdom. It shows how the NHS operates and helps migrant patients understand the differences from the healthcare systems they have been used to. There is also a link to an animated video explaining migrants' entitlements to NHS services in England, which can be used for interpreting practice.

Competences to be acquired: Interpreting and thematic/contextual competence.

3.2.3. Exercises to reinforce knowledge on cardiology

Cardiology 1 & 2, Learning Platform (<www.reactme.net/learning-platform/terminology>).

Outline: A series of exercises on the anatomy and physiology of the cardiovascular system and the meaning of terms relating to the heart.
Competences to be acquired: Medical and linguistic competence.

3.3. Week 3 (Cardiology – B)

3.3.1. Friday: History taking

A presentation should be prepared on how a patient's clinical history is taken using the SOCRATES method.
Outline: This presentation will help students to develop both their linguistic and medical competence and provide an insight into medical communication.
Competences to be acquired: Medical and linguistic competence.
<https://youtu.be/gsjKcQUsQY8>
Outline: Monolingual video of a nurse taking the clinical history of a diabetic patient. After interpreting the video into L2, students watch the video again to observe the SOCRATES method in action to understand the principles behind medical communication.
Competences to be acquired: Medical, linguistic, interpreting and interpersonal communication competence.
<https://youtu.be/9om2tedf9oo>
Outline: A second monolingual video, this time of a doctor speaking to a patient with chest pains for further interpreting practice into L2 and then to observe other ways in which doctors elicit information.
Competences to be acquired: Medical, linguistic, interpreting and interpersonal communication competence.

3.3.2. Saturday: Roleplay

Scripted bilingual roleplay with trainers playing both parts (not developed).

3.3.3. Introduction to codes of ethics

A presentation should be prepared to explain what a code of ethics is and why it is necessary in healthcare settings.
Outline: This presentation will analyse some codes of ethics (e.g. IMIA, CHIA, NCHIC codes of ethics), defining principles and strategies governing the conduct of members of this profession.
Competences to be acquired: Ethical and thematic/contextual competence.

3.3.4. Introduction to different types of roleplays

A presentation should be prepared to describe different types of structured roleplays in healthcare settings.
Outline: This presentation will describe scripted, unscripted and multi-role roleplays in healthcare.
Competences to be acquired: Interpreting, medical, linguistic and thematic/contextual competence.

3.3.5. Multi-role roleplay dealing with a case of angina

A presentation should be prepared on a specific heart disease like angina.
Outline: This multi-role roleplay will be focused on a case of suspected angina. In addition to the various specific symptoms and diagnostic tests, it should include some ethical dilemmas.
Competences to be acquired: Medical, linguistic, ethical and interpersonal communication competence.

3.4. Week 4 (Cardiology – C)

3.4.1. Friday: Cardiological examination and medical communication

<https://youtu.be/ECs9O5zl6XQ>
Outline: The video explains how a cardiac examination is performed. The doctor uses simple colloquial expressions to make himself understood,

always informing the patient what he's going to do in advance and asking the patient whether he has any questions. He then informs the patient of the diagnostic tests he will have to undergo (ECG, x-ray and blood tests).

Competences to be acquired: Interpreting, medical and medical communication competence.

3.4.2. Saturday: Interpreting practice

<https://youtu.be/8wdrG1Ct8og>
Outline: This monolingual video of a cardiological examination gives students further insights into the interactions between doctors and patients. Interpreting practice should be followed by an analysis of a further example of medical communication.
Competences to be acquired: Interpreting, medical, interpersonal and linguistic competence.
Multi-role roleplay in groups of 3 (not developed).
Outline: This multi-role roleplay should include some ethical dilemmas.
Competences to be acquired: Interpreting, medical, ethical, linguistic and interpersonal competence.

3.5. Week 5 (Orthopaedics – A)

3.5.1. Introductory texts

<https://my.clevelandclinic.org/health/articles/12254-musculoskeletal-system>
Outline: An easy-to-understand text on the musculoskeletal system, functions, anatomy, diseases and disorders.
Competences to be acquired: Medical and linguistic competence.
<https://youtu.be/zkcCPMzZDFo>
Outline: In this video from the Cleveland Clinic new orthopaedic imaging technologies and modalities are explained (3-D imaging, transplant imaging, CT-Scans, MRIs, etc.).

Competences to be acquired: Medical, interpreting, linguistic and information-mining competence.

3.6. Week B (6) Orthopaedics

3.6.1. Friday: Orthopaedic examination

<https://youtu.be/oh1G1-IycCw>
Outline: Monolingual video on an examination of the knee (Osce Guide). In addition to interpreting practice, this video of a doctor visiting a patient also provides a further example of medical communication.
Competences to be acquired: Medical, linguistic, interpreting and interpersonal competence.

3.6.2. Workplace knowledge

Presentation on the importance of workplace knowledge, such as the location of different departments in a hospital, the identification of hospital staff through their uniforms and their different roles.
Competences to be acquired: Thematic/contextual and information-mining competence.

3.6.3. Saturday: Interpreting practice

Interpreting of scripted bilingual roleplay involving an orthopaedic visit with trainers playing both parts performed in front of the class (not developed).

3.6.4. Intercultural issues

Presentation on intercultural issues, including topics such as pain and physical contact (not developed).

3.6.5. Interpreting practice

Multi-role roleplay in groups of 3 (not developed).
Similar materials to those provided for Weeks 1–6 can then be prepared following the indications given in the Guidelines and Module Programme.

Bibliography

Campbell, John. 2016. *Medical Terms 8, Cardiovascular, the Heart*. <https://youtu.be/nWRDYkB9IHU>.
Cleveland Clinic. n.d. *Musculoskeletal System*. <https://my.clevelandclinic.org/health/body/12254-musculoskeletal-system-normal-structure--function>.
Cleveland Clinic. 2013. *New Orthopedic Imaging Technology*. <https://youtu.be/zkcCPMzZDF0>.
Dirty Medicine. 2021. *Patient Centered Care & Breaking Bad News (SPIKES Model)*. <www.youtube.com/watch?v=cg2v97-9z9s>.
Drs Manual. 2019. *Chest Pain – OSCE History Taking for Medical Students*. <https://youtu.be/90m2tedf900>.
Gill, James. 2020. *The Cardiac Examination – Clinical Skills*. <https://youtu.be/ECs9O5zl6XQ>.
Hippocratix. 2017. *PASS THE CSA // MRCGP EXAM PRACTICE – Chest Pain // CSA Prep*. <https://youtu.be/8wdrG1Ct80g>.
Mayo Clinic. n.d. *Heart Disease*. <www.mayoclinic.org/diseases-conditions/heart-disease/symptoms-causes/syc-20353118>.
Nurseledclinics. 2012. *Master Clinical History Taking*. <https://youtu.be/gsjKcQUsQY8>.
Office for Health Improvement and Disparities. 2022. *NHS Entitlements: Migrant Health Guide*. <www.gov.uk/guidance/nhs-entitlements-migrant-health-guide>.
Quesmed. 2022. *Knee Examination – OSCE Guide*. <https://youtu.be/oh1G1-IycCw>.
ReACTMe. 2022a. *Terminology Exercises*. <www.reactme.net/learning-platform/terminology>.
ReACTMe. 2022b. *Training Resources Compilation*. <http://reactme.net/learning-platform/training-resources-compilation>.

UT Health San Antonio. 2013. *Delivering Bad News – An Excellent Encounter.* <www.youtube.com/watch?v=_uOS7hfKkVI>.

Warwick Medical School. 2016. *Clinical History Example – Using the Four Frames Approach.* <https://youtu.be/vlfdybUCzFw>.

WebMD Editorial Contributors. 2021. *Heart Disease: Types, Causes, and Symptoms.* <www.webmd.com/heart-disease/heart-disease-types-causes-symptoms>.

BEVERLY COSTA

7 Reflective Practice Support for Interpreters: Why, What and How?

1. Introduction

A mobile phone connects us to each other. Once its battery goes flat, it needs to be recharged or it will not be connecting anyone at all. The battery charger is one element of a circle of support which sustains and keeps the phone alive so it can continue to connect people. Interpreters also connect people together. But the cognitive and emotional load of the effort can make them go flat. Without some form of recharging how can they restore, revive, refresh or repair themselves?

In health and social care contexts spoken language interpreters[1] may be the voice that the patient hears telling them of a terminal diagnosis, the need for a limb to be amputated or the removal of a child into care. Not only are they the person a patient hears giving them life-changing information, but an interpreter also uses the first person 'I' to relay the patients' feelings and the intensity of those feelings to the clinician. And yet interpreters often feel that the practitioners for whom they interpret see them purely as a linguistic technician relaying messages in different languages (Hsieh 2008; Gryesten 2021). This differs from the view interpreters have of themselves. Interpreters believe they have a more complex

---

1   Although some of this chapter may be applicable to working with sign language interpreters, the reader may wish to refer to the NHS Guidelines for Working with British Sign Language/English Interpreters in Mental Health Settings (<www.rdash.nhs.uk/wp-content/uploads/2014/04/DP8403-Guidelines-for-working-with-BSL-01.19.pdf>) or the Association of Sign Language Interpreters (2020) for further information.

set of responsibilities and use a range of cognitive and affective skills to ensure that effective communication takes place between the different speakers. Interpreters may regard their profession as a profession of care, but they are expected to refrain from demonstrating this in mental health interventions (Gryesten 2021). This tension can result in the 'objectification of interpreters and their emotion work' by health workers (Hsieh and Nicodemus 2015: 1477). These professional differences in views and values can increase interpreters' stress.

Health and social care interventions are often emotionally demanding for practitioners. Research findings indicate that the work in healthcare takes an emotional toll on professions such as nurses (Li et al. 2014). Equally, work in health and social care can have an impact on interpreters who frequently have to deal with emotionally and ethically conflicting demands (Doherty 2010; Boyles and Talbot 2017; Hubscher-Davidson 2020).

Interpreters do a herculean job of managing their feelings in the moment. However, this often means that they do not have an opportunity to process those emotions. They also have very little room to manoeuvre in terms of their professional codes of ethics (Phelan 2019). And, as we have noted, healthcare practitioners can objectify interpreters. Interpreters can internalize this objectification and regard the pushing down of emotions as part and parcel of their job to be endured as if they were an object. Even if that were possible, it is counterproductive. Unprocessed emotions become lodged in the psyche. They continue to haunt us. The incremental effect of emotions being lodged and left unprocessed can have repercussions over days, weeks, and even years. And they can suddenly reappear when you least expect them. Here is a story and a metaphor to illustrate what I mean. A few years ago, I had to go to a formal function. I had put on weight, and I did not fit into the outfit I had bought for the event a few months previously. I put on some special stretchy underwear to try and flatten out some of the bulges. I got dressed and I asked one of my sons for his opinion. He said, 'Well that bit looks alright but that bit (he pointed to a bit that had not seemed so bad before) that bit's sticking out now.' And then he added some words that I have never forgotten. He said, 'Mum, the fat has got to come out somewhere.' That phrase stuck with me. Not just because you cannot hide it if you have put on weight (and why should you!), but because this is what happens when we squash our feelings down in an attempt to hide them. We do not deal with the feelings as they occur. Maybe we are too busy (focusing on the task of interpreting, for example) or the feelings are too painful, and we try to move away from them. They are stored not as a coherent narrative but as unprocessed traces and fragments of senses and emotions (van der Kolk 2014). But those squashed-down feelings have to come out somewhere, and they can come out when we least expect them. That is when they can cause damage, not only to ourselves but also to those around us.

In emotionally sensitive consultations clients show appreciation for interpreters' empathic engagement (Costa and Briggs 2014). However, empathic engagement (especially when empathy is enacted unconsciously) in emotionally charged situations can be draining over long periods of time. Unconscious empathy and compassion can impact negatively on physical as well as emotional well-being, while increasing the risk for compassion fatigue and vicarious trauma (Rothschild 2007). Harvey (2003) recognizes the negative effects empathic engagement can have on interpreters. He recommends that interpreters find ways to shield themselves from what he calls the 'perils of empathy'. Although he is referring to sign language interpreters, Harvey's observations can be applied to spoken language interpreters, who also work in an empathically engaged way.

To address the occupational stress experienced by interpreters a brief training intervention to train interpreters in a new role as interpreter-facilitators of Reflective Practice Groups was piloted between 2019 and 2022 by the Pásalo Project (<www.pasaloproject.org>). It was evaluated by twelve participating, qualified and experienced interpreters (ten with over fifteen years of experience) who completed an online anonymous questionnaire. The two most important outcomes identified were: learning about psychological safety; learning how to listen and to allow space for others to comment. Eight of the participants rated the course as highly effective in building their confidence to become an interpreter-facilitator of reflective practice/supervision groups. The pilot will be described later in the chapter.

2. Circle of support for self-sustainability

Let's think about the mobile phone again. Its battery charger can be viewed as one element, or segment, of a sustaining circle of support which enables the phone to continue connecting people to each other. Connection and empathic engagement with their clients require interpreters to invest emotional and cognitive energy, while containing their own emotional reactions. It is one segment of a circle of support and care. It is hard work, and it can wear you out. Support for interpreters forms another segment of the circle. Interpreters can access support to restore, revive, refresh and repair themselves. Giving and receiving support completes a circle. If the support comes from within the profession at the intraprofessional rather than interprofessional level, the circle of support can become self-sustaining.

Researchers, like Gieling et al. (2022), who study the stress on interpreters from working in sensitive contexts such as healthcare for migrants and refugees, recommend formal support structures for interpreters. Gieling et al. (ibid.) report on the results from 164 participants who responded to a survey about the psychological distress and trauma exposure related to working in refugee care in Germany. The results led the researchers to recommend that employers and interpreting agencies should offer supervision for interpreters.[2] This may also benefit interpreters who work in other care contexts.

Support for interpreters who work in healthcare is regularly recommended, but sadly, in present-day practice, it is seldom seen as a priority. Little has been written about the experience of running supervision groups for interpreters since two supervision groups for interpreters were described twenty-five years ago (Tribe 1997; Sande 1998).

---

[2] The researchers also recognize that this goes hand in hand with better pay and improved working conditions for interpreters.

3. What is supervision or reflective practice support?

As I mentioned earlier, squashed-down feelings have to come out somewhere. Support with difficult feelings is helpful not just because we appreciate feeling connected and not alone with our feelings, but also because the feelings are useful information. Reflective support helps us understand what it is that our feelings might represent. Feelings and emotional reactions can tell us things we might miss otherwise (Kurtz 2019). Although counselling or psychotherapy can be useful for individual personal healing and growth, support for one's occupation can often be more usefully delivered by what is called clinical supervision or reflective practice support. This is run by a trained facilitator. Clinical supervision or reflective practice support is not the equivalent of mentoring. It is not line management either, although the word supervision can be understood as a management function. There is no universally accepted definition of clinical supervision which distinguishes it from reflective practice support. Carroll (2007) offers a simple definition of supervision as a forum where supervisees review and reflect on their work in order to do it better. Both supervision and reflective practice support provide opportunities for repair, reflection and development and for the emergence of new responses to difficult situations. Reflective practice support is a form of support used regularly by professions such as psychology, psychotherapy, social work and counselling. It provides an opportunity, and a safe and confidential space, to process emotions and to help to make sense of them so that we make good decisions in the moment. Schön (1983) calls this 'reflection-in-action'. Kurtz (2019: 4) describes reflective practice in groups as an opportunity 'to develop the capacity of the group to use peer support and create a more reflective working culture'. For interpreters, who frequently work in isolation, a group format may be very welcome as a form of support as well as the chance to learn from each other.

I prefer to use the term reflective practice support or reflective support for interpreters rather than supervision to avoid confusion. Framing supportive reflective practice as continuous professional development may also make its purpose even clearer if this is a new experience for interpreters.

4. How is reflective practice support delivered?

Reflective practice support is not viewed as an expendable option by many of the caring professions. Practitioners are expected to commit to attend sessions on a regular basis, not just when there is a pressing need or a crisis. Support groups typically meet regularly once a month. The commitment to ongoing support is important. This is about ongoing self/group care even when things seem to be going OK. Because 'going OK' does not always accurately represent the incremental effect of unprocessed emotions. Reflective support is not about a quick fix for a crisis. It is about being there for your colleagues as well as being there for yourself.

Of course, there is a question about who pays for this support. This is an especially pertinent question for freelance interpreters whose work is not ongoing but intermittent. O'Connor (2022), who reports on her research about the supervision needs of arts practitioners working in health and social care, suggests that it is the responsibility of the organizations who employ them to provide this support, possibly within the framework of continuous professional development. These suggestions are equally valid for the interpreting profession.

Reflective practice support is reparative, personally and professionally developmental, and it has the capacity to transform practice (Kurtz 2019). Reflective support takes places individually or in groups. As already mentioned, support in groups can be welcomed by interpreters who often work on their own for long periods.

Reflective groups do not have a set agenda. Their effectiveness is driven by the material that members of the group are willing to bring to discuss. The conversations are based on a model of reflective practice which considers *what* we know (through our felt sense as well as through our cognition) and *why* we know it. The kinds of material interpreters bring to a reflective practice support group (RPSG) include experiences from an interpreting assignment that may have left them with a lot of feelings and emotions; a situation where they had to make an ethical decision; a concern that they may be burning out or becoming vicariously traumatized through their empathic engagement which may cause them to have symptoms which are

Reflective Practice Support for Interpreters

similar to their traumatized clients. Interpreters may have a general question, concern or observation they wish to share with the group, and they want to hear group members' thoughts about it. The following is a range of examples of issues and questions that might be discussed. They are an amalgamized and anonymized selection of questions and issues that interpreters have raised in RPSGs I have run for the past twenty years. They represent different health contexts. Some of the examples relate to asylum and trafficking contexts, while other examples are less specifically situated:

> I had to interpret for a 14-year-old girl. She is pregnant because she was raped by the agent who brought her here. I can't stop thinking about her.
>
> I interpreted for a teenage boy who kept shouting and saying he was going to kill himself. I don't know what happened to him. I am not sure if he is alive.
>
> The practitioner refused to give me a briefing meeting.
>
> A patient was really rude and said I was too young to interpret for him.
>
> I was interpreting for a patient who says he hates all Africans. But I am African. What should I do when a client is prejudiced or is acting in a discriminatory way? It affects me.

5. Ethical issues

In a reflective practice group, confidentiality is held within the group. All the members of the group commit to refrain from discussing or commenting outside of the group on any of the material they hear about through participating in the group. Interpreters, who are bound by strict guidelines about confidentiality in their interpreting work, can therefore feel free and safe to bring concerns or issues from their work that are troubling them or that they find challenging or interesting. Members of the group also commit not to judge or criticize. As a group they strive to work together to find creative solutions to challenges. However, it is important to recognize that all the members of the group are responsible for their own work. They each have a duty of care towards their clients, and they are ultimately responsible for the resolution of any difficulties they encounter. A facilitator would not normally take any action that affected an individual group member's practice. They would only contact a member's professional body in the unlikely case of unresolved unprofessional practice. Facilitators of reflective practice are also required to have reflective supervision of their own facilitation of others.

6. Facilitation of reflective practice groups: A new role for interpreters?

Support groups for interpreters tend to be facilitated at the interprofessional level by clinicians such as psychological therapists. Psychological therapists are often trained in supervision skills, and they may also have experience of running personal and professional development groups. Some interpreters may appreciate the opportunity to participate in support groups facilitated by clinicians. However, interpreters who have found themselves in groups facilitated by clinicians with little or no experience and training in working with interpreters can find the experience frustrating.

To facilitate RPSGs clearly requires sensitivity, skills and awareness of the ethical challenges of personal and professional development work. However, it could be argued that designating the position of facilitator of interpreter's support interventions to clinicians maintains the power dynamic and the hierarchical structure of interpreter-mediated healthcare where interpreters occupy a passive position with limited agency. Although it is appropriate for clinicians to lead the consultation in a healthcare context, why does this dynamic need to be repeated in the reflective practice context? This concern, in addition to the issue of clinicians facilitating interpreter groups who are inexperienced in working with interpreters, could be addressed by training interpreters in reflective practice group facilitation skills. Once trained, the facilitators would also be expected to continue with ongoing supervision of their facilitation of reflective practice groups.

Such an initiative – training non-clinicians to facilitate intraprofessional supervision – is not without precedent.

A project developed by the British Association for Counselling and Psychotherapy (BACP 2021) offers reflective practice supportive supervision skills training for teachers. The BACP model is a training course to upskill staff in educational settings to provide and receive peer-to-peer supervision (Holmes and Page 2021). The model provides an illustration of training non-clinicians to become reflective practice support facilitators in a self-sustaining way. Likewise, training interpreter-facilitators enables support for interpreters to be intraprofessional and to be self-sustaining.

7. Training interpreter-facilitators

Some initiatives to train interpreters to facilitate peer-to-peer support and reflective support groups are already taking place. These include projects such as the '360 Supervision' Diploma in Supervision for Sign Language Interpreters (<https://360supervision.co.uk>) and the Pásalo Project's (<www.pasaloproject.org/trainingconsultancy.html>) interpreter-facilitation training in collaboration with the Association of Interpreters and Translators (UK) (Facebook/AIT.professionals) and community interpreting organizations in Scotland and Wales. Facilitating reflective practise support groups is not specifically within interpreters' skill sets. However, many interpreters' skills are transferable and their professional skill sets can be developed and expanded (Hewson and Carroll 2016). The following example comes from a programme developed by the Pásalo Project.

The programme of training prepares interpreters to run reflective support groups for their fellow interpreters. The training initiative is based on an apprenticeship/learning-by-doing model (Vygotsky 1978; Kolb 1984; Gibbs 1988; Collins et al. 1991) and an approach which dismantles and makes visible participants' 'knowing-in-action' (Schön 1983). These active learning approaches build on interpreters' skills and encourage them to put their adapted skills into practice from day one of the training, with practical homework tasks between sessions and four follow-up practice sessions after the three-day training programme has been completed.

All participants take part, as active participants, in RPSG sessions facilitated by the trainer. After each session, everyone – participants and trainer – deconstructs and discusses the process of the group facilitation which the trainer has modelled. The competencies and skills that a facilitator of a RPSG for interpreters needs to develop are drawn out from participation in the group and the post-participation discussions about the process. The trainer is questioned about their rationale for decisions they have made when they were facilitating the group sessions.

7.1. Example of the apprenticeship/learning-by-doing model (based on an amalgamized and fictionalized situation)

A group of eight interpreters are attending a three-day training course to learn how to facilitate a RPSG. It is day one of the course and, as an introduction to learning about how to create a psychologically safe space for a group, they take part in a RPSG facilitated by Hywel, the course trainer. During part of the RPSG one member of the group, Soraya, tells a story about a difficult ethical dilemma she faced.

The trainees are active participants in the RPSG, and they are all asked simultaneously to observe the behaviour and decisions made by Hywel. The trainees make notes on Hywel's behaviour, actions and attitudes. When the group session finishes, Hywel invites the trainees to offer feedback to him about the skills and competencies they witnessed, or that they thought were missing, in his performance. What has Hywel done that the trainees have found helpful and what have they found not so helpful? What did Hywel do that contributed to their feeling psychologically safe/unsafe in the group? Do they have any questions for Hywel about the decisions he made during the facilitation of the session?

*When the trainees have made some general observations, one trainee, Paulo, asks Hywel a question about his instruction to the group. After Soraya had told her story Hywel asked the group to share their own thoughts and feelings but **not** to ask Soraya further questions. Paulo said it felt strange and he also felt a bit annoyed at not being able to ask Soraya anything else. He asks Hywel why he instructed them not to ask questions. Hywel shares his rationale for this. One of the reasons, he explains, is to allow the 'sharer' – in this case, Soraya – some space and to release her from the spotlight. The 'sharer' may feel quite vulnerable and isolated after sharing. Now it is the 'sharer's' time to receive something back from the group without anything else being required of them. This is* *an opportunity for the rest of the group to reach out and connect with the 'sharer.' After everyone in the group, who wanted to, had spoken, Soraya had the opportunity to respond to what she had heard. She also had the chance to have the last word. Hywel goes on to explain the psychological thinking behind these decisions and their relevance for the concept of a safe psychological space in a group.*

The content from the session that has just been described could have been taught in a lecture format. However, the learning-by-doing approach allows the group to feel the impact of the facilitator's behaviour and to discover for themselves how safety in a group can be created. The learning-by-doing approach requires that, if any essential skills and competencies have not been addressed in the discussion phase, the trainer completes any gaps in the observations to ensure that all the competencies and skills needed to facilitate a RPSG for interpreters are covered. These competencies and skills include: learning how to create a psychologically safe space; encouraging discussion of ethical issues; containing participants' anxiety and fear of being judged; self-awareness and management of your and others' emotions, communicating and intervening appropriately; engaging, modelling and encouraging intelligent empathy; navigating appropriately the 'support–challenge' continuum; facilitating conversations about difficult issues; giving and receiving feedback appropriately; pre-empting, identifying and managing possible triggers for participants; noticing parallel processes, facilitating the cycle of experiencing/learning/applying to practice.

During the three days of training participants practice peer support and they also practice facilitating a reflective support group for interpreters. At the end of the three-day course participants organize four practice group sessions so that they can continue to practise running groups without the trainer present. After each of the four practice groups the trainer provides group supervision for the facilitator(s) of the groups.

The training programme provides a comprehensive practical introduction to reflective facilitation skills, which is further embedded by ongoing supervision of facilitation practice.

8. Interpreter-facilitation: A post-training example of practice

Pásalo Project has delivered interpreter-facilitator training to three organizations including In-Trans (<www.in-trans.co.uk>) interpreting and translating service of the Grampian Regional Equality Council (GREC). One outcome from the training at In-Trans GREC is the provision of a RPSG for new and inexperienced interpreters who have been recruited quickly, with little time for induction as a result of the large numbers of Ukrainian refugees from the war in Ukraine settling in Aberdeen. The sudden events of war and other catastrophes can mean that interpreters have to be recruited and trained very quickly. The RPSG is facilitated by one of the 'graduates' from the interpreter-facilitator training programme. The RPSG was presented as continuous professional development and is attended by five interpreters who are all deployed in the emergency Ukrainian resettlement programme. When the groups were originally conceptualized, it was envisaged that interpreters with varying language profiles and repertoires would attend and that the groups would be run by facilitators communicating in English as the lingua franca. In this group, however, as the interpreter-facilitator is a Russian speaker, there was the possibility of communicating in Russian. Despite political sensitivities, the group has requested to be able to use both Russian and English in the group for which there is great appreciation.

9. Conclusion

The cumulative nature of emotional demands on interpreters in health and social care contexts and their need for appropriate support have been well documented. Mental health professionals, nurses and social workers are required to attend regular reflective supervision in order to recharge their emotional batteries, to maintain the standard of their work and to complete the circle of care. Even if it is not currently a requirement for interpreters, reflective practice support is recommended for them. It would have the same benefit for them as for other professionals. When you engage empathically with another person, your own feelings and emotions are switched on. You may switch them off in the moment, but they do not just go away. They have to come out somewhere.

RPSGs can provide an effective form of support for interpreters with those feelings and emotions that otherwise can continue to haunt them. Such groups are a form of support that interpreters can be trained to deliver. A learning-by-doing approach to the training builds on their skill set so that they can reach an appropriate ethically safe level to practice in a relatively short period of time. Anecdotal evidence suggests that interpreters who have participated in a group facilitated by a trained interpreter-facilitator feel understood and well-supported. They appreciate the facilitator's interpreting experience as well as their ability to offer parts of the session in different languages. Additionally, some interpreters perceive training to become a reflective practice group facilitator as a career progression route. Ultimately, it would be ideal if the training programme for interpreter-facilitators of reflective practice groups could be offered and accredited by universities and colleges.

Appropriate support breathes life back into a deflated practitioner as the supporter is supported. The 'container' is 'contained' (Bion 1962). Teaching interpreters to run RPSGs for themselves completes interpreters' circles of support – from giving to receiving and then learning how to support others – so that they can continue with their work as an integral and essential element of the health and social services' circles of support and care.

RPSGs are like the battery charger for a mobile phone. They can help interpreters to recharge their emotional and cognitive batteries. Trained interpreter-facilitators of the groups make the system self-sustaining.

Bibliography

BACP. 2021. 'Reflective practice supportive supervision skills training'. <www.bacp.co.uk/news/news-from-bacp/2021/reflective-practice-supportive-supervision-skills-training>.

Bion, Wilfred R. 1962. *Learning from Experience*. London: Heinemann.

Boyles, Jude, and Nathalie Talbot. 2017. *Working with Interpreters in Psychological Therapy*. London: Routledge.

Carroll, Michael. 2007. 'Coaching psychology supervision: Luxury or necessity?', in Stephen Palmer and Alison Whybrow (eds), *Handbook of Coaching Psychology: A Guide for Practitioners*. Hove: Routledge, 431–448.

Collins, Allan, John S. Brown, and Ann Holum. 1991. 'Cognitive apprenticeship: Making thinking visible', *American Educator: The Professional Journal of the American Federation of Teachers* 15(3), 6–11 and 38–39.

Costa, Beverley, and Stephen Briggs. 2014. 'Service-users' experiences of interpreters in psychological therapy: A pilot study', *International Journal of Migration, Health and Social Care* 10(4), 231–244. <https://doi/10.1108/IJMHSC-12-2013-0044>.

Doherty, Sharon M., Anna M. MacIntyre, and Tara Wyne. 2010. 'How does it feel for you? The emotional impact and specific challenges of mental health interpreting', *Mental Health Review Journal* 15(3), 31–44.

Gibbs, Graham. 1988. *Learning by Doing: A Guide to Teaching and Learning Methods*. Oxford: Oxford Further Education Unit.

Gieling, Angelika, Christine Knaevelsrud, Maria Böttche, and Nadine Stammel. 2022. 'Psychological distress, exhaustion, and work-related correlates among interpreters working in refugee care: Results of a nationwide online survey in Germany', *European Journal of Psychotraumatology* 13(1), 1–12. <www.tandfonline.com/doi/full/10.1080/20008198.2022.2046954>.

Gryesten, Jasmin R., Kathrine J. Brodersen, Laura G. Lindberg, Jessica Carlsson, and Stig Poulsen. 2021. 'Interpreter-mediated psychotherapy – a qualitative analysis of the interprofessional collaboration between psychologists and interpreters', *Current Psychology: A Journal for Diverse Perspectives on Diverse Psychological Issues* 42, 1420–1433. <https://doi.org/10.1007/s12144-021-01345-y>.

Harvey, Michael A. 2003. 'Shielding yourself from the perils of empathy: The case of sign language interpreters', *Journal of Deaf Studies and Deaf Education* 8, 207–213. <https://doi.org/10.1093/deafed/eng004>.

Hewson, Daphne, and Michael Carroll. 2016. *Reflective Practice in Supervision*. New South Wales: MoshPit.

Holmes, Joanna, and Stephen Page. 2020. 'How pastoral workers in Further Education are benefiting from supervision', *BACP University and College Counselling* 9(3), 23–28.

Hsieh, Elaine. 2008. '"I am not a robot!" Interpreters' views of their roles in health care settings', *Qualitative Health Research* 18(10), 1367–1383. <https://doi.org/10.1177/1049732308323840>.

Hsieh, Elaine, and Brenda Nicodemus. 2015. 'Conceptualizing emotion in healthcare interpreting: A normative approach to interpreters' emotion work', *Patient Education and Counselling* 98, 1474–1481. <https://doi.org/10.1016/j.pec.2015.06.012>.

Hubscher-Davidson, Severine. 2020. 'Ethical stress in the translation and interpreting professions', in Kaisa Koskinen and Nike K. Pokorn (eds), *The Routledge Handbook of Translation and Ethics*. Abingdon: Routledge, 415–430.

Kolb, David. A. 1984. *Experiential Learning: Experience as the Source of Learning and Development*. Englewood Cliffs: Prentice-Hall.

Kurtz, Arabella. 2019. *How to Run Reflective Practice Groups: A Guide for Healthcare Professionals*. Abingdon: Routledge. <https://doi.org/10.4324/9781351112994>.

Li, Angela, Sean F. Early, Nicole E. Mahrer, Jessica L. Klaristenfeld, and Jeffrey I. Gold. 2014. 'Group cohesion and organizational commitment: Protective factors for nurse residents' job satisfaction, compassion fatigue, compassion satisfaction, and burnout', *Journal of Professional Nursing* 30(1), 89–99. <https://doi.org/10.1016/j.profnurs.2013.04.004>.

O'Connor, Alison. 2022. 'The work hurts', *Journal of Applied Arts & Health* 13(2), 153–166. <https://doi.org/10.1386/jaah_00096_1>.

Phelan, M., Rudvin, M., Skaaden, H., and Kermit, P. 2019. *Ethics in Public Service Interpreting*. 1st edn. Abingdon: Routledge. <https://doi.org/10.4324/9781315715056>.

Rothschild, Babette. 2007. *Help for the Helper-the Psychophysiology of Compassion Fatigue and Vicarious Trauma*. New York: Norton Professional Books.

Sande, Hans. 1998. 'Supervision of refugee interpreters: 5 years of experience from northern Norway', *Nordic Journal of Psychiatry* 52, 403–409.

Schön, Donald A. 1983. *The Reflective Practitioner: How Professionals Think in Action*. London: Temple Smith.

Tribe, Rachel. 1997. 'A critical analysis of a support and clinical supervision group for interpreters working with refugees located in Britain', *GROUPWORK* 10(3), 196–214.

Van der Kolk, Bessel. 2014. *The Body Keeps the Score: Brain, Mind, and Body in the Healing of Trauma.* New York: Viking Press.

Vygotsky, L. S. 1978. *Mind in Society: The Development of Higher Psychological Processes.* Cambridge, MA: Harvard University Press.

CYNTHIA E. ROAT

8 Reweaving the Tapestry: How Healthcare Interpreters Will Save the World[1]

1. Introduction

I am honoured to be invited to address you today, from the other side of the world in Seattle, WA. When I was invited to speak at the ReACTMe final conference and to contribute to this volume, we discussed what I should address. I thought about discussing the consequences of a lack of clear communication in health care, such as a patient's inability to share their health history, a provider's inability to accurately diagnose, the resulting overuse of unnecessary diagnostic tests, the lack of patient compliance to treatment plans, and poor health outcomes both on the community and individual level. But you probably know about these already. Next, I thought about discussing how trained interpreters can improve the quality of communication in health care, leading to improved access to care, improved quality of care, increased patient safety and lower costs of care. But you most likely already know about this as well. Finally, I thought I would reflect on the great work accomplished by the ReACTMe project, which has not focused on problems in language access but on comprehensive and sustainable solutions to those problems. But the readers of this volume will know better than anyone what the ReACTMe team members have already accomplished.

So instead, I am going to discuss what lies ahead. While the completion of the ReACTMe project marks an important highpoint, this is not

---

1   The contents of this chapter were presented as a keynote address to the final international conference of the ReACTMe project on 21 July 2022.

the end of the road. There is much left to do. The ReACTMe team members are educators, and they have accomplished a wonderful educational goal. They are like farmers who have grown the perfect radish. If, however, they cannot get those radishes to market, to a cook and onto the dinner table, they have not achieved their true goal. In the same way, if their well-trained interpreters are not serving regularly in hospitals and clinics across the country, what will they have gained?

So, how does that happen? How do trained interpreters get integrated into the healthcare system? If you will allow me, I would like to share some experiences from the past thirty years of building language access programmes in the United States. I do so not in the spirit of telling you what you should do, because our situations are all different, but in the spirit of sharing with colleagues an experience, hoping that something in there might be of use to you as you move forward. To do this, I have to tell you a bit about what language access for spoken languages was like in the United States in 1990.

2. Language access in the United States in 1990

In the early 1990s in the United States, very few healthcare facilities had any formal strategy for providing interpreter services. It was not uncommon for patients who spoke limited English to be told that they needed to bring their own interpreter, and family or friends – with all their attendant limitations – provided the bulk of the language services. Sometimes untrained self-assessed bilingual staff was called upon to interpret. In only a very few places were minimally trained dedicated interpreters made available. For the most part, communication with Limited English Proficient (LEP) patients was substandard at best.

This ad hoc approach to dealing with language barriers should not be surprising. There was no public financial support to pay for interpreters, and very little research to show that interpreters would make a difference in either quality of care or health outcomes. Telephonic interpreting was in its infancy – very expensive and not widely adopted – so interpreters had to be on site for even the shortest encounter. And while there was a legal requirement (Title VI of the 1964 Civil Rights Act) for recipients of federal funding to provide interpreters, most healthcare facilities were unaware of these requirements, and only the Office for Civil Rights of Region X (the Pacific Northwest) had provided guidance to recipients in their region of their responsibilities to provide language access. Finally, it must be mentioned that language services were seen as a benefit primarily to the patients, who were Native Americans, refugees or immigrants: all underserved communities generally seen as uninsured and unimportant.

To make matters worse, those of us working for language access were all functioning in silos. Remember, this was before the internet. Advances were being made in Boston, in Minneapolis, in Seattle, but there was only sporadic and informal communication between those involved. There were no interpreter associations that addressed the concerns of healthcare interpreters specifically. Within the language professions, diplomatic, conference and court interpreters commonly viewed their colleagues that worked in health care as being 'not real interpreters'. And how could we argue otherwise? There was very little training available specifically for healthcare interpreters, and this only in a few places. Most of these courses were under 15 hours of instruction, and we did not even require proof of bilingual language proficiency to register. As for certification of healthcare interpreters, there was none.

In summary, in the early 1990s, healthcare interpreting in the United States was in its infancy. Today, the field has reached adulthood. Well, all right, maybe adolescence. How did we get from there to where we are now? The field did not move ahead in large jumps, but rather in an upward spiral of small improvements that led to more small improvements over time. Here are some of the strategies that moved the field forward over the past thirty years.

3. Strategies used in the United States

3.1. The carrot and the stick

Convincing hospitals and clinics to provide paid interpreters has required a combination of 'carrots' and 'sticks'. The carrot has been the clear superiority of trained, qualified interpreters in facilitating understanding in communication between patients and providers speaking different languages. The stick has been legal action against facilities that fail to provide adequate language access.

Let's look at Seattle, for example. In the late 1970s, in the aftermath of the Vietnam War, healthcare facilities in the city found themselves providing care to a refugee population with serious healthcare needs and with languages and cultures that few mainstream providers had previously encountered. Vietnamese, Cambodian, Lao and Hmong were among the languages suddenly being heard in clinics and hospitals across the city. Several community clinics responded by training and employing Southeast Asian medical assistants, who also served as (albeit untrained) interpreters. In the early 1980s a larger group of community clinics serving immigrant and refugee populations procured a grant to form the Community Health Interpretation Service (CHIS) to provide a pool of shared interpreters for their various clinics. This system worked well, until the patients were referred to specialists or to inpatient care, where they received no language services at all. So CHIS began to provide interpreters for free to the hospitals. Providers began to notice the difference between the trained medical interpreters from CHIS and the ad hoc interpreters they had to work with otherwise. In 1981, the Health Department and three hospitals agreed to split the salary of one staff interpreter to serve all three hospitals. One interpreter for three hospitals was clearly inadequate, still, the hospitals were unwilling to do more. The carrot had run its course; it was time for the stick.

Finally, legal advocates in Seattle filed a formal complaint with the Department of Health and Human Services Office for Civil Rights (OCR), alleging that these three hospitals had violated their LEP patients' civil rights by neglecting to provide equal access to care. They followed up with legal suits. In short order, the hospitals signed a contract with CHIS to provide 24/7 coverage. By 1995, this programme was serving over 20 hospitals in 40+ languages and with over 150 on-call interpreters (Wilson Owens and Jackson 2003).

It may be that the civil rights complaint alone might have forced the hospitals into providing interpreters. However, combining the 'stick' of legal action with the 'carrot' of the positive relationship built with CHIS and the positive experience of providers with the trained interpreters made the transition from ad hoc language services to routine language services smoother and more palatable to hospital administrators.

3.2. Improving research

Healthcare is a field ruled by empirical data. While to many, it may seem that being able to clearly communicate with one's patients would be an obvious benefit in the provision of health services, the lack of research regarding the need for and impact of interpreter services made it difficult to convince hospital administrators to add a significant expense to their already overtaxed budgets. In the late 1990s and early 2000s, however, an upsurge in serious research started to document the impact of language barriers on health outcomes (Chan et al. 2005), the impact of the provision of trained interpreters on quality of care (Bard et al. 2004) and cost of care (Bernstein et al. 2002), and the experiences of LEP patients and providers with and without interpreters. With each additional study, advocates had more empirical data to share with dubious administrators, and the stronger the argument for engaging trained interpreters. In 2003, The California Endowment commissioned an annotated bibliography of studies regarding language access in health care (Jacobs et al. 2003) in order to make this research more easily accessible to mid-level managers and interpreter advocates, who used it to good effect. As hospitals started to hire a few interpreters, usually Spanish, these began to collect data within their respective hospitals on patient demographics, demand for interpreters, and the hospitals' ability (or inability) to meet the demand. This data could then be used to build a case for hiring additional interpreters. There is no doubt that the development of a research literature on the need and impact of language access, linked to data from individual hospitals, played a significant role in the expansion of many language access programmes.

3.3. Legislation

It is clear that legislation has played a significant role in advancing language access in the US Enforcement, however, is the key. Title VI of the Civil Rights Act, prohibiting discrimination based on race, colour or country of national origin, was made law in 1964. The US Supreme Court ruled in 1974 that language was an aspect of 'country of national origin' (Lau v. Nichols 1974). However, in 1990, only a few hospitals around the United States were in compliance. It was not until the federal Department of Health and Human Services (DHHS)' Office for Civil Rights began to actively investigate complaints based on national origin discrimination that change really started to happen. Between 1990 and 2003, DHHS received 122 complaints about failures to provide language access. In 2002, DHHS finally published a national LEP Guidance, similar to the regional guidance emitted by its Region X office in 1989, detailing the responsibilities of recipients of federal funding in providing language access (US Federal Register 2000). DHHS even started to conduct proactive compliance reviews of major medical centres, giving teeth to the Civil Rights Act and making Title VI more of a reality.

Unfortunately, changes in federal administrations impacted the degree to which the Office for Civil Rights (OCR) continued to actively enforce Title VI. Under politically liberal administrations, OCR tended to investigate complaints of national origin discrimination more aggressively; under conservative administrations, these complaints went to the bottom of the pile. This situation, and the slow pace of civil rights investigations, limited the degree to which Title VI could be effectively applied.

Other federal statutes, however, as well as federal regulations, state laws, managed care contracts and tort liability also addressed the problem of limited language access. In 2003, the National Health Law Program, a national public law organization, published a 200+ page compendium of all the legal measures affecting language access in the United States (Wilson-Stronks and Galvez 2007).

In 2010, the US Congress passed the Patient Protection and Affordable Care Act. Section 1557 of this Act enshrined and expanded the prohibitions against discrimination guaranteed in the 1964 Civil Rights Act (Patient Protection and Affordable Care Act 2010). Language access advocates took this opportunity to help shape rules implementing Section 1557 that clearly spelled out healthcare institutions' responsibilities to provide not only interpreters, but qualified interpreters. These provisions were weakened under the Trump administration but are being once again restored under the Biden administration.

3.4. Accreditation

In the United States, hospital administrators pay attention when the Office for Civil Rights comes calling. But when The Joint Commission (TJC) is at the door, the entire hospital jumps. Healthcare institutions in the United States must be accredited in order to receive any kind of federal funding, such as Medicaid (public insurance for low-income people) or Medicare (public insurance for the elderly and disabled). The largest organization accrediting healthcare institutions in the United States is TJC. TJC accredits member hospitals every three years, and hospitals pay very close attention to the standards TJC applies. To lose accreditation effectively means to close the doors.

In 2007, TJC completed a three-year study of sixty hospitals in the United States with regard to language access (Wilson-Stronks and Galvez 2007). As a direct result of this study, the Commission started in 2008 to require accredited hospitals to track patients' language preferences. In 2010, new standards were adopted that directly required the free provision of interpreter services and documentation as to how interpreters' qualifications were ascertained (Joint Commission on Accreditation of Healthcare Organizations 2010). Arguably, this change in accreditation standards did more to focus hospitals' attention on language access than any of the legal pressures.

3.5. Funding

Who's going to pay for all this? Whether public or private, healthcare institutions in the United States are almost universally non-profit organizations and are all under immense financial pressure. So, when the Region X Office for Civil Rights reminded recipients of federal funds in the Pacific North-west in 1989 that they had to provide interpreters, hospitals and clinics protested that it was an 'unfunded mandate' which they could not afford. Clinics that accepted Medicaid, which traditionally reimburses providers less than the cost of care to begin with, began to threaten to stop serving Medicaid populations at all if they had to pay for an interpreter. In the end, Washington State found a clever way to use part of the Medicaid funding it received from the federal government to pay for interpreters for patients on Medicaid. This move was a great help to hospitals and clinics, and other states followed suit. However not all states did; due to the convoluted way in which healthcare is financed in the United States, some states found it was not to their benefit to use their Medicaid dollars this way. In those states, interpreter services are still funded by each hospital's operating budget. This funding issue is one with which we are still struggling.

3.6. Engaging the press

How do we create public support for language services when the public is often unsupportive of the very patients who need those services? The press can be a tremendous ally in this fight. During the 1990s and 2000s, major newspapers such as *Newsday* (Cheng 2003), *The New York Times* (Bernstein 2005), and *Ft. Lauderdale's Sun-Sentinel* (De Aztlan 2006) began to run stories about the difficulties faced by immigrants who could not communicate with their doctor until an interpreter arrived to save the day. They covered court cases in which hospitals were sued because of tragic outcomes linked to an unmet need for an interpreter (Lee 2007). These articles helped raise public awareness and made people think about what it would be like to seek health care in a language they did not understand. Such articles also put pressure on hospitals seeking to avoid bad publicity and instead establish a good reputation in their communities.

Engaging the press, however, can also backfire. At times, the advocates who called the press were successful in getting hospitals to make changes. However, the hospitals were understandably unwilling to engage the whistle-blowers, whom they saw as antagonistic, as advisers. As a result, sometimes the experts who could have best helped hospitals improve were excluded from helping to solve the problems.

3.7. Learning to speak the language

In 1995, I gave my first presentation on language access to a group of hospital leaders in Atlanta, Georgia. In my best social-reformer voice, I lectured them on the social injustice of not providing interpreters and on the risk that they would be sued or that the Office for Civil Rights would investigate them. They actually laughed at me. Legal challenge, they told me, was unlikely to come from disempowered groups such as immigrants and refugees. And the OCR in Georgia was so busy investigating complaints based on racial discrimination that they would never get around to looking into national origin complaints. I had entirely missed the mark. More to the point, I was speaking to them in a language they did not understand. As an interpreter, I should have known better!

Over the years, however, many of us in the language access field have learned the language of the decision makers in health care. To the Chief Executive Officers, we talk about The Joint Commission and patient safety. To the Chief Financial Officers, we talk about how interpreters could save them money. To doctors, we underscore how interpreters could make their jobs easier and lead to better patient outcomes. We save the social justice arguments for community activists.

3.8. Changing norms

In the 1990s, I was frequently asked by hospital administrators, 'Why do we have to provide interpreters?' However, as the year 2000 rolled around, I started hearing a different question from administrators: 'How can we provide language access most efficiently?' And in 2008, the Chief Executive Officer (CEO) of a Managed Health Care Plan in California responded when I asked him about cutting the interpreter service as a means of containing costs, 'Cut the interpreters? Are you crazy – how would we communicate with our members?'

Sometime between 1990 and 2008, a shift had occurred in the norms of providing health care. Whereas in 1990, discussions about language access and interpreting were limited to small groups of advocates outside of healthcare administration, by 2008, the topic was being addressed openly in conferences and publications from the American Medical Association (Tanya 2001), the National Association of Public Hospitals (1995) and the California Academy of Family Physicians (Roat 2005). In 1990, most Interpreter Service departments existed outside the hospital administrative framework and were responsible for raising their own budget, managing their own personnel issues, and handling their own information technology (IT). By the mid-2000s, these departments were part of the hospital, like any other department, folded into the operating budget, with access to the hospital's Human Resources Department and IT support. Somewhere along the way, language access had ceased to be an ad hoc activity and became part of the standard set of services provided by the hospital.

4. Lessons for Europe?

As I said at the start of this chapter, I do not share our experiences in the United States in order to provide a roadmap for Europe. Each of you, as individuals and as countries, will find your own road. However, could any of our experiences in the United States be instructive in some way?

Might there be opportunities to create grant-funded interpreter collaboratives that could start providing trained interpreters to hospitals so that providers would come to appreciate the difference that a trained interpreter can make?

Are there laws in European countries that could be used to pressure hospitals that are unwilling to take seriously the linguistic needs of their immigrant and refugee patients? If health care is considered in your country to be a basic human right, could that be used to your advantage? Who are your natural allies among those who champion the rights of migrants?

Are you familiar with the research literature around language access and interpreting? Here I am not referring to the literature around training interpreters, which is also important, but the body of research showing how trained interpreters effect quality of care, patient safety, health outcomes and cost of care. Does research done in the United States have any credibility in your country, or does research need to be done locally so that it applies more directly?

Do you know what most concerns your hospital administrators? Your healthcare providers? Can you speak their languages when you talk to them? Who will your champions be from the ranks of the doctors and hospital administrators?

Are your healthcare institutions accredited? If so, by what body? Do those accrediting institutions look at language access? If not, how could they be made to consider that aspect of care?

Funding will always be a central issue. How can you be creative in helping to set up systems that are efficient, matching modality to need, perhaps creating a tiered qualification for interpreters, with more advanced interpreters earning more? Could technology help connect patients and providers with interpreters in languages of lower demand, or for shorter appointments, as a means of lowering costs and making it easier to get an interpreter?

How do you garner public support for these programmes? What does the press in your countries have to say about immigrants and refugees? Can you find stories about individuals and families that your communities would find sympathetic and compelling?

If the provision of language services is not the norm today in your healthcare systems, what would change those norms? Which are the conferences, or the publications, or the modes of communication through which healthcare administrators and providers need to hear about these issues? How can you get access to those?

Think back to the upward spiral that I mentioned in the previous pages. What are small steps you can take immediately? If starting a whole interpreter programme is too much, what about finding a grant to start a small pilot programme? If a large research study is intimidating, what about collecting demand and usage data at one clinic? If hospitals refuse to hire interpreters, what about offering your most advanced students to do internships, which would benefit them, the hospitals and the patients? If changing federal law is too onerous, what about introducing legislation supporting language access in your town or province?

And finally, what other levers might be effective in your country, in your hospitals, in your communities? In Japan, for example, the pressures of the upcoming 2020 Olympics in Tokyo led to the designation of certain hospitals as 'tourist hospitals' where interpreters would be provided and to the expanded training of interpreters. An upsurge in medical tourism in the country also led to an increased interest in having trained interpreters available. Each country has its own particular situation and motivators. What are yours?

4.1. Hold on just a minute!

I hear you all out there, shouting, 'Just hold on a minute! We are interpreters! We are educators! We are researchers! There is no way we can do all this!' No, you cannot, not you alone. But you are not alone.

You – interpreters and educators – build the profession. Researchers provide data and studies to push the agenda. Physician champions and mid-level managers build systems to engage interpreters. Community advocates and the press create external pressure on hospitals. Entrepreneurs create the marketplace to normalize the provision of interpreter services.

Reweaving the Tapestry

There are many players on this team, which means you had best get started on your networking.

4.2. The need will not go away

The need for the interpreters is only going to grow. A quick look at census data in the United States shows an ever-increasing number of LEP individuals, arriving as immigrants or refugees, learning English at a rapid pace but still needing interpreters in health care.[2] Clinicians reference a shift from acute to chronic illness in our populations, management of which requires understanding of the condition and therapy, life-style changes and follow-up, all of which require clear and repeated communication. Everywhere we see the growth of technology-mediated care such as telemedicine and patient-provider messaging through web portals, which depend entirely on communication. And health care is focusing increasingly on care coordination and patient safety, both of which are communication dependent. Because of all of this, in the United States, the Bureau of Labor Statistics forecasts that the translation and interpreting professions will grow 20 per cent from 2021 to 2031, much faster than the average for all occupations (US Bureau of Labor Statistics 2022).

But we also see cuts to interpreter services budgets. We see a shift to using exclusively remote modalities with no consideration of the nature of the appointment. Healthcare administrators still seem to underestimate both the need for interpreters and the difficulty of the work. And, of course, we are still struggling against a small, very vocal segment of the population that harbours strong anti-immigrant sentiment. Finally, we have to ask ourselves if human interpreters will be replaced soon with automated interpreting apps run by artificial intelligence. The need for language services is not going away, but the form in which those services are provided may be changing significantly.

---

2   US Census data show that the number of individuals who report speaking English 'less than very well' in the United States rose from 14 million (6.1 per cent) in 1990 to 21.3 million (8.1 per cent) in 2000 to 27 million (8.2 per cent) in 2020.

5. Conclusion

I do not think, however, that machines can take the place of human interpreters. When I started in this field thirty years ago, I had a dream – a dream that anyone could walk into a hospital in the United States and, regardless of the language they spoke, access healthcare as easily as if they spoke fluent English.

It meant changing the entire way in which health care would be delivered across languages. We are not there yet, but we are closer than we were in 1990. And what keeps me going in this work, what stops me from tossing my computer out the window or kicking certain doctors in the shins, is remembering why we do this.

Consider something that I was told by Mr Thomas June, a Mandarin and Cantonese interpreter in Seattle in 1995. Mr June observed:

> When a refugee walks into our hospital, everything is strange. The sights are strange. The smells are strange. The sounds are strange. There is only one familiar thing in all this strangeness – the voice of the interpreter.

I see our world being torn apart by global crises that could hardly have been imagined a few generations ago: global warming, increasingly destructive wars, growing disparities between the rich and the poor. So often, the reaction to these threats is principally fear. I see people seeking security in the known and the familiar, as the division between 'us' and 'them' becomes more common first in our individual thoughts, then in our interpersonal relationships, then in our institutions, and even in our national politics. Because 'they' are different, foreign, incomprehensible. To paraphrase Mr June, they look different, they smell different, they sound different. Imagine the doctor attempting to treat a patient who the doctor cannot understand, whose very words and interactions are so foreign that the doctor cannot build the patient-provider relationship on which effective healthcare depends. Every individual encounter like this leaves a tiny rent in the fabric of our societies, and as these small rips run into each other, the tapestry of society becomes tattered, riddled by gaping holes, starting to unravel. The result is that the hopeful trends toward unity at the local, national and international levels during the late twentieth and early twenty-first centuries seem to have stalled, foundered, and started to backtrack into rampant nationalism, isolationism, and violence.

Except – there it is – the voice of the interpreter. As Mr June said, it is to the patient the only familiar thing in all this strangeness. And to the doctor, the interpreter becomes the means by which this incomprehensible patient suddenly starts to sound familiar. The doctor thinks, 'This mother is concerned about the same things that last patient worried about! This pattern of symptoms is easily diagnosed!' The patient agrees to the treatment plan because she can now understand the doctor, trust the doctor and trust the treatment plan. And both doctor and patient leave the encounter feeling connected instead of alienated.

And so, little by little, in hundreds of thousands of short encounters in health care and social service venues across the continent, community interpreters are quietly, carefully, unobtrusively mending the rips in the fabric of our communities. Your work to recruit and to train interpreters, to engage providers and build language access programmes, is a phenomenal act of education, but not just of education. It is a phenomenal labour of social justice. Of turning the 'them' into 'us'. There is no more important piece of work in the world today.

This is why I am honoured to contribute to this volume. ReACTMe, and all of you reading this, have taken on a huge task, but you are ready for it. I rejoice to know that, in the years to come, the interpreters formed by your programs, in Romania, in Italy, in Spain, in whatever country you inhabit, will be out there, every day, quietly and unobtrusively reweaving the tapestry of your communities, one interpretation at a time.

Bibliography

Bard, Michael R., Claudia E. Goettler, Paul J. Schenarts, Beth A. Collins, Eric A. Toschlog, Scott G. Sagraves, and Michael F. Rotondo. 2004. 'Language barrier leads to the unnecessary intubation of trauma patients', *The American Surgeon* 70(9), 783–786. <https://pubmed.ncbi.nlm.nih.gov/15481294>.

Bernstein, Nina. 2005. 'Language barrier called health hazard in E.R.', *The New York Times*, 21 April. <www.nytimes.com/2005/04/21/nyregion/language-barrier-called-health-hazard-in-er.html>.

Bernstein, Judith, Edward Bernstein, Ami Dave, Eric Hardt, Thea James, Judith Linden, Patricia Mitchell, Tokiko Oishi, and Clara Safi. 2002. 'Trained medical interpreters in the emergency department: Effects on services, subsequent charges and follow-up', *Journal of Immigrant Health*, 4(54), 171–176. <https://pubmed.ncbi.nlm.nih.gov/16228770>.

Chan, Kitty S., Emmett Keeler, Matthias Schonlau, Mayde Rosen, and Rita Mangione-Smith. 2005. 'How do ethnicity and primary language spoken at home affect management practices and outcomes in children and adolescents with asthma?', *Archives of Pediatrics & Adolescent Medicine* 159(3), 283–289. <https://jamanetwork.com/journals/jamapediatrics/fullarticle/485953>.

Cheng, Mae M. 2003. 'Need seen for interpreters at hospitals', *Newsday*, 25 November.

De Aztlan, Toni. 2006. 'The language Rx: Health care for many immigrants would be lost in translation if not for the emerging presence of medical interpreters', *Sun-Sentinel (Fort Lauderdale, Florida)*, Broward Metro Edition, 13 August.

Jacobs, Elizabeth A., Niels Agger-Gupta, Alice Hm Chen, Adam Piotrowski, and Eric J. Hardt. 2003. 'Language barriers in health care settings: An annotated bibliography of the research literature', *The California Endowment*. <https://ncihc.memberclicks.net/assets/documents/cal.endow.bibliography.pdf>.

Joint Commission on Accreditation of Healthcare Organizations. 2010. *Joint Commission Perspectives* 30(1).

Lau v. Nichols, 414 US 563. 1974. See Lau v. Nichols: 414 US 563 (1974): Justia US Supreme Court Center.

Lee, Seok Ho. 2007. 'Family blames lack of medical interpreters in young woman's death', translated by Aruna Lee, *Korea Times* 19.

National Association of Public Hospitals. 1995. *Agenda of the 1995 Annual Conference of the NAPH in Santa Fe, New Mexico*.

Patient Protection and Affordable Care Act, Section 1557. <www.hhs.gov/civil-rights/for-individuals/section-1557/index.html>.

Roat, Cynthia E. 2005. 'Addressing language access issues in your practice: A toolkit for physicians and their staff members', *The California Academy of Family Physicians*. <www.healthdesign.org/sites/default/files/CalEndowment_language_access_issues.pdf>.

US Bureau of Labor Statistics. 2022. *Interpreters and Translators: Occupational Outlook Handbook*. <www.bls.gov/ooh/media-and-communication/interpreters-and-translators.htm>.

Wilson Owens, Christine, and J. Carey Jackson. 2003. '*Collaborative Strategies for Language Access in Health Care in Seattle & King County* [Meeting Report].

Refugee and Immigrant Health Promotion Program at Harborview Medical Center. <https://ethnomed.org/wp-content/uploads/2020/01/Collaborative-Strategies-For-Language-Access-In-Health-Care-In-Seattle-King-County.pdf>.

Wilson-Stronks, Amy, and Erika Galvez. 2007. *Hospitals, Language and Culture: A Snapshot of the Nation*. The Joint Commission and The California Endowment. <www.kyha.com/assets/docs/QualityDocs/EffectiveCommunications/jointcommissionpaper.pdf>.

ANA ISABEL FOULQUIÉ RUBIO

Annex. Guidelines for Working with Medical Interpreters

Sometimes, healthcare professionals are not used to work with interpreters and this presents a challenge for them. At the same time, professional interpreters have to face the challenges of working with other professionals who do not know much about their role and the way interpreting works.

These guidelines are based on the experiences and opinions gathered mostly in the workshops organized with healthcare students and professionals and on the experience of researchers within the ReACTMe project. The idea is to disseminate this information using different means such as the project webpage. These guidelines will also be available in the different languages with their own QR code.

These guidelines include the following ten points and their respective short explanations:

1. Brief interpreters
Interpreters work in different medical settings, so the more information they get, the better they perform.

2. Allow interpreters to introduce themselves
Not everybody is used to working with interpreters, so allow interpreters to explain their role to both you and the patient whenever possible.

3. Suggest where they should stand/sit
Everything that happens is important as regards communication, so please consider that interpreters need to be able to hear and, preferably, also see everything that happens.

4. Speak directly to the patient – NOT to the interpreter
In order to promote direct communication with your patient, avoid requests such as 'tell/ask him/her'.

5. Remember that interpreters translate everything that is said

Therefore, avoid saying anything that you don't want to be translated and never ask the interpreter to summarize information or finish quickly.

6. *Speak clearly and pause frequently*

Even when interpreters take notes, they can only memorize a certain amount of information and may need to ask for repetitions or clarification.

7. *Check for understanding*

Make sure that the patient has received the information you wanted to convey by using checking questions.

8. *Never leave interpreters alone to give medical explanations*

As a healthcare professional, you must always be present during the interpreted consultation.

9. *Debrief the interpreter after the patient has left (whenever possible)*

Even a few minutes can help you and your interpreter improve future interpreted consultations.

10. *Remember that the interpreter is an ally.*

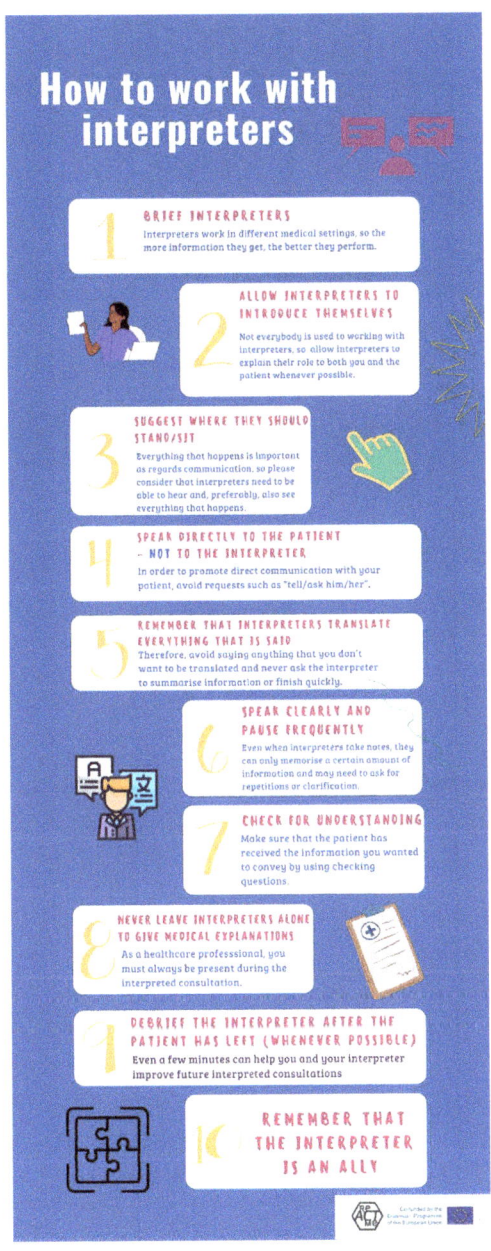

Figure A.1. English guidelines for working with medical interpreters

Figure A.2. Spanish poster with QR code to access guidelines for working with medical interpreters

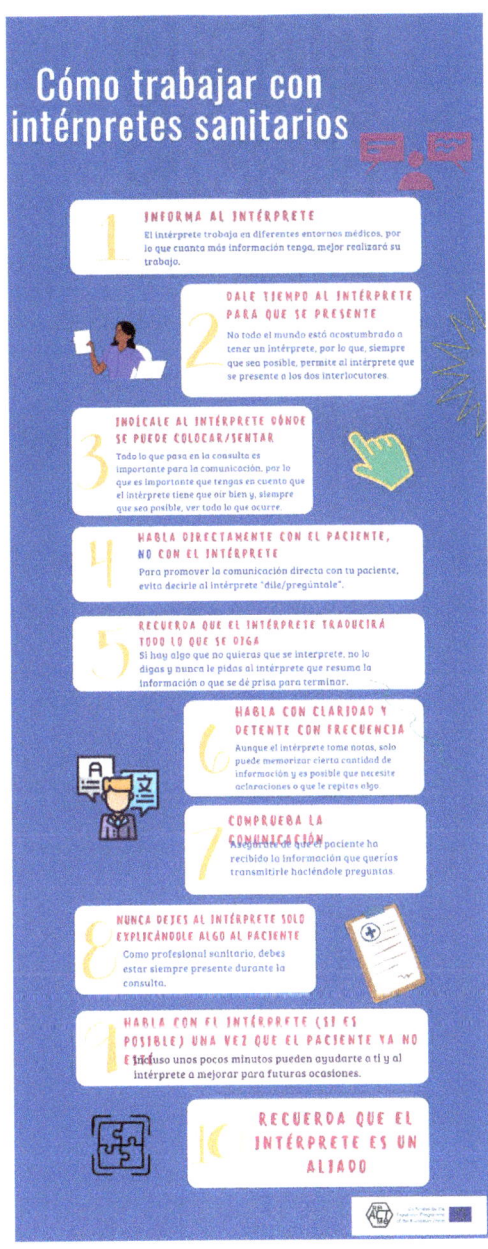

Figure A.3. Spanish guidelines for working with medical interpreters

Figure A.4. Italian poster with QR code to access guidelines for working with medical interpreters

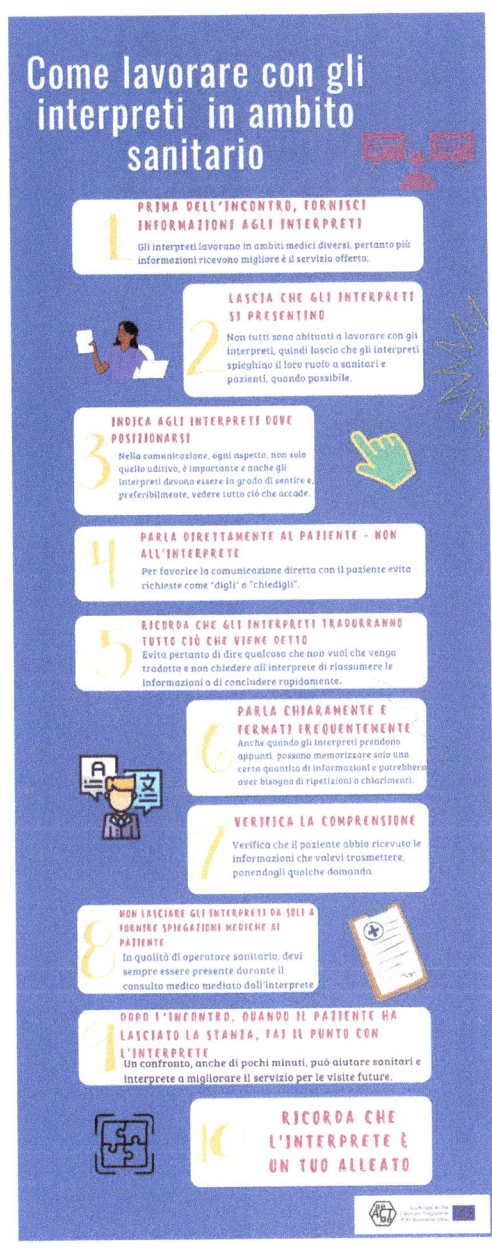

Figure A.5. Italian guidelines for working with medical interpreters

Figure A.6. Romanian poster with QR code to access guidelines for working with medical interpreters

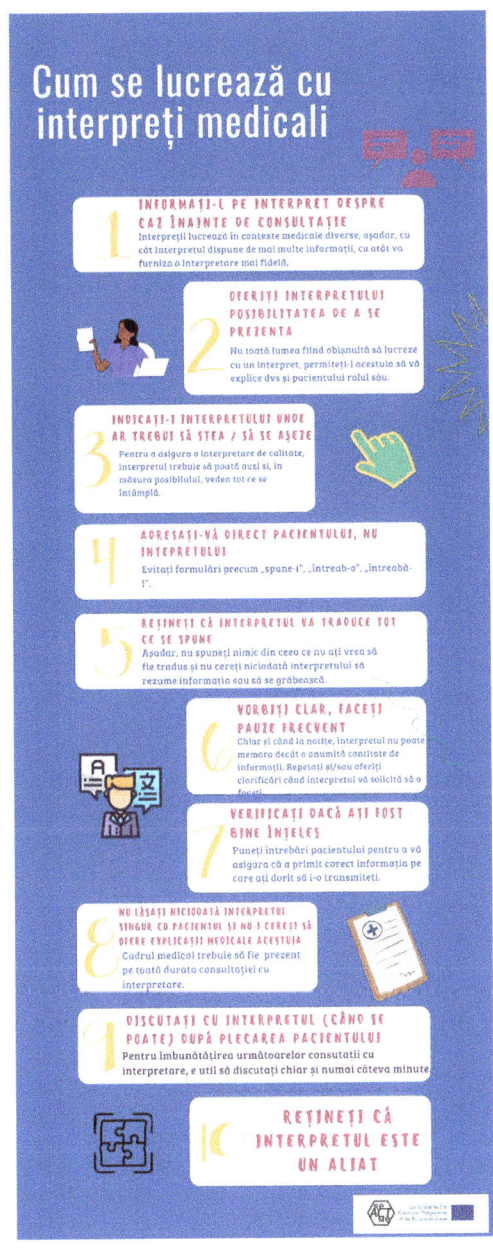

Figure A.7. Romanian guidelines for working with medical interpreters

Notes on Contributors

ALINA ANDREICA is a Lecturer in the Department of Modern Languages at 'Iuliu Haţieganu' University of Medicine and Pharmacy, Cluj-Napoca, Romania, where she teaches Romanian as a Foreign Language for general and medical purposes to international students; designs and publishes teaching materials; conducts Romanian language testing; and organizes tandem teaching and learning. She holds a master's degree in Multicultural Studies and a doctoral degree in Philology, both from Babes Bolyai University, Romania. Her research interests include Romanian as a Foreign Language, Romanian for Specific Purposes, medical terminology, language immersion, multilingualism, alterity, and literary folklore

ELEONORA BERNARDI is a professional conference interpreter working in the Institutional and private sector with Italian, English, French and Croatian as her working languages. She also served, from 2013 to 2017, as a resident medical interpreter at the hospitals of Rimini and Riccione, Italy. After having worked as a contract professor and a lecturer at the University of Bologna and at the University of Macerata, she is currently completing her PhD in interpreting at Bologna's Department of Interpreting and Translation (DIT).

LINDSEY BRUTON is a lecturer at San Jorge University (Spain) where she teaches both English for specific purposes in the field of health sciences and language teaching pedagogy. She is also responsible for language testing and assessment at the university, coordinating and teacher training for both internal and external language evaluation. She has participated in the design and implementation of the university's language policy and internationalization programme largely within the area of CLIL (Content and Language Integrated Learning) teacher training and support. Lindsey is currently involved in several European projects relating to Innovation in Education and learning and has published articles and book chapters relating primarily to this field and centring on Internationalization, CLIL, assessment, critical thinking and gamification.

DONATELLA CIFOLA holds a master's degree in European and American Languages and Literatures, a bachelor's degree in Modern Languages and Literature, and a diploma in Interpreting and Translation (English, German and French). Since 2014, she has been Adjunct Professor in Dialogue and Consecutive Interpreting (German–Italian) at UNINT- Università degli Studi Internazionali, where she also teaches extracurricular courses of Medical-Pharmaceutical Language (English, French, German). From 2000 to 2012, she was a lecturer at Università degli Studi di Perugia (Italy) within several departments, mainly in the Department of Medicine, where she taught English to nurses and healthcare professionals. She works as a freelance interpreter and translator. Her research interests focus mostly on Translation and Interpreting Studies, the impact of globalization on languages, medical and pharmaceutical translation and interpreting and international relations.

BEVERLEY COSTA trained as a psychotherapist and then set up Mothertongue multi-ethnic counselling service (2000–2018) for multilingual clients. In 2009 she created a pool of mental health interpreters and in 2010 she established the national Bilingual Therapist and Mental Health Interpreter Forum and founded The Pásalo Project in 2017 <https://www.pasaloproject.org/> to disseminate learning from Mothertongue. In 2013, Beverley established 'Colleagues Across Borders' offering support to refugee psychosocial workers and interpreters based mainly in the Middle East and Eastern Europe. She is a Senior Practitioner Fellow at Birkbeck, University of London and has written multiple papers and chapters. Beverley has produced a play about a couple in a cross-language relationship for the Soho Theatre, London. Her book *Other Tongues: Psychological Therapies in a Multilingual World* was published in 2020. She created the online training resource on multilingualism and mental health in 2021/22 <https://www.pasaloproject.org/multilingualism-mental-health-and-psychological-therapy---course-content.html>.

ANA ISABEL FOULQUIÉ RUBIO holds a PhD in Translation and Interpreting from the University of Murcia, an Undergraduate Degree in Translation and Interpreting from the University of Granada, and a Master's Degree in Alien Law. Currently she is a full-time lecturer of Translation and Interpreting at the University of Murcia, where she is responsible for teaching Public Service Interpreting, amongst other courses. She participated in the creation of the Research Group, GRETI of the University of Granada, and currently belongs to the Research Group TRADICO of the University of Murcia. She has participated in different research projects such as 'Conceptualization and Assessment of Creativity in Translation' (funded by the Seneca Foundation) and 'EMOTRA, Translation and Emotions' (funded by the Spanish Ministry of Education) and the ReACTMe Project (funded by the European Commission). She has worked as a freelance translator and interpreter for twenty years. She has published articles and chapters mainly related to public service interpreting.

CHRISTOPHER GARWOOD is a conference interpreter and Research Fellow at the University of Bologna, where he has been a conference and dialogue interpreter trainer for almost thirty years at the Department of Interpreting and Translation (Forlì). He has also organized and taught in numerous courses and seminars on interpreting in various fields, in particular in the legal setting. His research has focused above all on the teaching of interpreting, with several publications on this topic.

FRANCESCA GNANI is an Adjunct Professor at Università deli Studi Internazionali in Rome, where she teaches Medical Interpreting and Medical Translation in BA and MA courses, respectively. She has twenty years of experience as a freelance interpreter and translator and she is member of AITI (Italian Translators' and Interpreters' Association). She published a paper on the impact of Covid on medical interpreting in Italy in 2022. She joined the ReACTMe team in 2019.

VERONICA MANOLE is a lecturer at the Faculty of Letters of Babeș-Bolyai University (Romania). She is the coordinator of the BA Programme in

Portuguese Studies and of the Camões Portuguese Language Center in Cluj-Napoca. She received her PhD in 2015 from Paris VIII University, after defending a thesis on Portuguese, Brazilian, and Romanian parliamentary discourse. She has published extensively on discourse analysis, pragmatics and inter-comprehension in Romance languages, being one of the six authors of the textbook *PanromanIC, manuale di intercompreensione fra lingue romanze*. She is also a conference interpreter, active on the Romanian market and was a member of the ReACTme project.

ALMUDENA NEVADO LLOPIS holds a PhD in Translation, Society and Communication from Jaume I University (Spain). She is a full-time lecturer in Undergraduate Degrees in Translation and Nursing, and the Master's Degree in Research for Health Sciences at San Jorge University (Spain). She belongs to the research group Migrations, Interculturality and Human Development (MIDH). She has participated in several international research projects, such as Sino-European interculturality, valorizing and professionalizing knowledge in institutional and marketing communication and TC Nurse Transcultural Nursing. From 2019 to 2022, she coordinated the Erasmus+ project Research & Action and Training in Medical Interpreting (ReACTMe). Almudena has researched and published in the fields of intercultural communication, public service interpreting, medical interpreting and intercultural mediation.

NATACHA NIEMANTS is Associate Professor at the Department of Interpreting and Translation of the University of Bologna (Italy), where she teaches French-Italian conference and dialogue interpreting. Her research interests include interpreting in healthcare and asylum-seeking contexts, interpreter training, transcription, and conversation analysis. She has published papers in books (John Benjamins, Lambert-Lucas, L'Harmattan, Peter Lang) and international journals (ELA, Interpreting, InTRAlinea, Langage et Société, Meta), is author of *L'interprétation de dialogue en milieu médical: Du jeu de rôle à l'exercice d'une responsabilité* (Aracne, 2015), and in collaboration with Letizia Cirillo she has edited *Teaching Dialogue Interpreting. Research-based proposals for higher education* (John Benjamins, 2017). She has also collaborated to the *Routledge Encyclopaedia of Interpreting Studies* (Pöchhacker ed. 2015) with an entry on transcription and has recently joined the Editorial Board of *The Interpreters' Newsletter*, after guest-editing two issues on dialogue interpreting in 2015 and 2021.

ALINA PELEA holds a PhD in Translation Studies (Babeș-Bolyai University and University of Artois). She is a lecturer at the Department of Applied Modern Languages of the Faculty of Letters, Babeș-Bolyai University, where she teaches conference interpreting and French grammar. She is the coordinator of the MA in Conference Interpreting in the same department and her research currently concerns mainly interpreting training, and medical interpreting, but also the cultural and sociological aspects of interpreting and literary translation. The main results in her research on literary translation were published in the volume *La Traduction: crapaud ou Prince charmant?! Aspects culturels de la traduction du conte merveilleux* (Casa Cărții de Știință, 2020). From 2019 to 2022, she coordinated the ReACTMe team at Babeș-Bolyai University. She also works as a freelance interpreter and translator.

CYNTHIA E. ROAT, MPH, is an interpreter trainer and language access consultant based in the United States. Certified as a medical and social-service English–Spanish interpreter, she interpreted in a wide range of community settings in the early 1990s, before her interest in systems change led her into training interpreters, instructors, medical providers and healthcare administrators. Over the past three decades, Ms Roat has made significant contributions, both in the United States and abroad, as a consultant, researcher, author, organizer and mentor. She is known as an engaging speaker, a knowledgeable resource, and an energetic advocate for language access in general. More information about Ms Roat's contributions to the field can be found on her website at <www.cindyroat.com>.

ELENA TOMASSINI obtained a Conference Interpreting Diploma (1980) and Degree (2004) at SSLMIT, University of Trieste, Italy. She has been working as conference interpreter since 1980 and is a member of Assointerpreti. She has specialized in medical conferences and has worked in several other sectors such as cinema, food and wine, environment, etc. She has been working as Conference and Dialogue Interpreting Adjunct Professor since 1992, first at SSLMIT, Forlì, UNIBO, and then at FIT (Faculty of Interpreting and Translation), UNINT, Rome, and other universities. She participated in the EU Erasmus+ Project 'Nursing on the Move' as developer, after working on the 'Medics on the Move' Leonardo da Vinci projects. She coordinated the UNINT ReACTMe research team. She co-wrote a book with Mette Rudvin, *Interpreting in the Community and Workplace: A Practical Teaching Guide* (Palgrave MacMillan, 2011), and has published some articles on medical interpreting.

Index

access to healthcare 15, 18, 30 *see* access to healthcare (services) 15, 20, 40, 74
accreditation 2, 6, 105, 111, 207 *see* accreditation procedures 121 *see* accreditation standards 207–208
accuracy 28, 36, 140
activities 20, 86, 111, 141, 146, 161, 163
    ad hoc 210
    learning 146
    linguistic 147
    multilingual 146
    preparatory 160
ad hoc interpreters 1, 28, 29, 34, 35, 41, 43, 44, 45, 46, 48, 50, 86, 93, 103, 104, 118, 204 *see also* children 36, 43, 104, 118 *see also* family 1, 11–13, 34, 35, 36, 43, 104, 118, 202 *see also* friends 1, 11–13, 29, 32, 35, 43, 97, 104, 106, 118, 202 *see also* non-professional interpreters 1, 6, 11–12, 32, 99, 124 *see also* relatives 32, 35, 36, 41, 43, 44, 97, 106
allophone patients 1, 2, 3, 4, 10, 16, 18, 26, 28, 40, 47, 48, 50, 96, 103, 104
associations 4, 10, 11–13, 14, 22, 33, 51, 59, 86, 87, 103, 104, 105, 114, 115, 117, 119, 124, 203
    American Medical Association (AMA) 210
    Asociación Española de Traductores, Correctores e Intérpretes (ASETRAD) 114
    Asociación de Intérpretes de Conferencia de España (AICE) 114
    Asociación Internacional de Traductores y Redactores de Medicina y Ciencias Afines (TREMEDICA) 114–115
    Asociación Profesional de Traductores e Intérpretes Judiciales y Jurados (APTIJ) 114
    Asociaţia Profesională a Interpreţilor şi Traducătorilor (APIT) 116
    Association of Sign Language Interpreters 185
    Association of Interpreters and Translators (UK) 193
    Associazione Internazionale di Interpreti di Conferenza (AIIC Italia) 115
    Associazione Italiana Traduttori e Interpreti (AITI) 115
    Associazione Nazionale Italiana Traduttori e Interpreti (ANITI) 115
    Associazione Nazionale Interpreti di Conferenza Professionisti (ASSOINTERPRETI) 115
    British Association for Counselling and Psychotherapy 193
    International Association of Conference Interpreters (AIIC) 105
    National Association of Public Hospitals (NAPH) 210
    UNI 23, 87
    Uniunea Naţională a Traducătorilor şi Interpreţilor din România (UNTAR) 116

asymmetry 87, 90, 164
asynchronous *see* asynchronously 150, 156, 172
   learning 134, 149, 155, 156, 157
   materials 166
   training 148
   work 135
awareness 3, 6, 25, 35, 36, 49, 50, 51, 76, 90, 97, 104, 105, 107, 116, 120, 134, 192, 209 *see* self-awareness 195 *see* emotional awareness 90

bachelor's (BA) degrees 58, 59, 106 *see* bachelor's courses 59
bilingual staff 44, 104, 202
Blended Intensive Program (BIP) 110

California Academy of Family Physicians (CAFP) 210
cardiology 134, 135, 136, 145, 148, 158, 167, 168, 169, 175, 176, 177, 178, 179
caregivers 45
case studies 5, 128, 133, 134, 137, 138, 139, 148, 149
certification xii, xiii, 2, 23, 105, 111, 113, 115, 120, 130, 203
   bodies 84
code of ethics 11, 24, 54, 121, 179, 186
communication
   intercultural 59, 62, 65, 68, 75, 81, 91
   interpersonal 164, 174, 178, 179
   medical 140, 168, 169, 178, 179, 180, 181
Community Health Interpretation Service (CHIS) 204
comparative analysis 14, 16, 20, 21, 49, 57, 58, 61
compassion fatigue 187
competences xiii, 4, 5, 11, 16, 23, 26, 28, 60, 61, 67, 83, 84, 91, 92, 94, 128, 129, 131, 132, 137, 138, 141, 142, 143, 148, 149, 153, 154, 158, 161, 165, 167, 174, 175, 176, 177, 178, 179, 180, 181
   cultural and intercultural 129, 130, 132, 138, 153, 174, 176, 181
   instrumental and professional 129, 130, 131
   interpersonal 129, 130, 131, 138, 153
   psychophysiological 129, 131, 132, 138
   strategic 129, 130, 131, 141, 142
   thematic xiii, 68, 83, 129, 130, 131, 142, 149, 153, 175, 176, 177, 179, 181
confidentiality 25, 28, 48, 90, 95, 120, 191
continuous professional development 77, 189, 190, 196
Conversation Analytic Role-Play Method (CARM) xiii
corpus xiii *see* corpora xiii
   analysis xiii
   tools xiii
courses 5, 23, 32, 40, 58, 59, 60, 61, 62, 64, 67, 68, 69, 70, 71, 72, 74, 75, 76, 77, 78, 86, 89, 90, 91, 96, 97, 103, 104, 105, 106, 107, 108, 109, 110, 120, 142, 150, 153, 154, 156, 157, 203
cultural barriers 1, 2, 11, 12, 23, 29, 31, 35, 86
cultural presuppositions 35
curriculum 2, 77, 127, 152, 154 *see* curricula 57, 58, 59, 75, 76, 77, 86, 89, 94, 106
cyclical structure 157

data collection 10 *see also* data-collection method 10
database 69, 129, 131
decalogue 6
decentralization 28, 29
decision makers 2, 3, 10, 11, 12, 13, 14, 33, 60, 91, 94, 209 *see also* policy/

decision makers 2, 3, 10, 11–13, 33, 60, 91, 94, 209
degrees 58, 61, 69, 76, 78, 85, 86, 106, 108, 123
Department of Health and Human Services Office for Civil Rights (DHHS OCR) 204
didactic units 134, 135, 136
discrimination 2, 20, 24, 206, 207, 209
doctors 12, 21, 27, 29, 31, 33, 34, 35, 36, 37, 39, 41, 43, 45, 46, 85, 88, 90, 93, 94, 95, 115, 118, 148, 160, 161, 168, 178, 180, 209, 211, 214
doctor-patient interactions xiii, 90
document analysis 4, 10, 58, 60, 77
documentation skills xiii

education xii, 23, 58, 59, 69, 89, 128, 150, 215
  higher 2, 3, 4, 57, 60, 91, 94, 134, 137, 144, 145, 146, 150
  higher institutions 2, 75, 104, 153
  interprofessional xiii
effectiveness 190
elective course 92, 109
emergency 45, 123
  care 58
  cases 30
  department 38, 39, 41, 90, 116
  room 134, 145
  services 38, 43
  situations 90, 116, 117
  surgery ward 39
emotional
  awareness 90
  batteries 196, 197
  burden 118, 123, 175
  demands 196
  energy 188
  impact 83, 92, 108
  implications 82
  involvement 94, 121
  labour
  load 105, 185
  maturity 88
  reactions 188, 189
  situations 87, 175
  support 5
  toll 186
  well-being 187
emotionally sensitive 187
empathic engagement 187, 188, 190
English as a lingua franca 46, 48
equality 2, 18
ethical
  challenges 135, 142, 192
  codes 93, 114
  commitment 130
  competence 174, 176, 179, 180
  decisions 190
  dilemmas 93, 132, 138, 168, 172, 173, 179, 180, 194
  guidelines 60, 89, 93, 138, 140
  issues 92, 93, 105, 109, 158, 161, 164, 191, 195
  nature 105
  norms 130
  practice 51
ethics xiii, 13, 72, 75, 107, 108, 113, 168 *see also* code of ethics 11, 24, 54, 121, 168, 174, 179, 186
  committee 10
European norms 112
European Observatory of Health Systems and Policies 18
expectations 4, 9, 21, 25, 26, 27, 28, 35, 57, 60, 72

face-to-face 134, 141, 155, 157, 166
  contexts 146
  learning 134
  lessons 156

mode 150
training 132, 149, 150
facilitators 5, 187, 192, 193, 196, 197
focus groups 4, 57, 60, 61, 82, 83, 84, 85, 87, 88, 89, 91, 92, 93, 94, 95, 96, 97, 108, 109, 119, 120
foreign-language speaking patients 1, 11, 12, 60
formal support 188
formal training in medical interpreting 57

gatekeeping 36
glossaries 5, 91, 116, 117, 129, 134, 136, 149
  see also multilingual glossaries 5, 129, 134, 136, 149
guidelines 2, 5, 6, 17, 27, 60, 89, 90, 93, 112, 136, 138, 140, 153, 156, 182, 191, 219, 221, 222, 223, 224, 225, 226, 227

heads of hospitals 21, 26, 32
healthcare
  professionals xiii, 4, 6, 11, 12, 13, 14, 25, 29, 30, 32, 34, 35, 36, 37, 38, 39, 40, 42, 45, 47, 48, 60, 83, 84, 91, 92, 93, 96, 97, 103, 104, 107, 109, 111, 115, 118, 119, 122, 124, 133, 150, 155, 161, 175, 219
  providers (HCP) 1, 3, 9, 10, 11, 12, 21, 34, 37, 83, 118, 140, 174, 211
  services 2, 4, 10, 12, 13, 15, 17, 18, 19, 20, 21, 26, 35, 40, 44, 61, 66, 68, 74, 85, 93, 95, 97, 115, 123, 124, 130
  systems 15, 16, 49, 83, 167, 175, 177, 212
  users (HCU) 9, 12, 21, 24, 40, 44, 47
history taking 83, 168, 169, 171, 172, 178
hospitals 5, 10, 17, 19, 20, 21, 23, 26, 29, 30, 31, 32, 34, 38, 41, 44, 45, 46, 47, 48, 49, 50, 71, 88, 89, 95, 105, 107, 109, 110, 116, 117, 118, 119, 120, 122, 144, 145, 170, 175, 181, 202, 204, 205, 206, 207, 208, 209, 210, 211, 212, 214

improvements xii, 21, 37, 39, 47, 48, 50, 105, 109, 116, 120, 124, 150, 203
in-house interpreters 30, 105, 117
informed consent 24, 29, 37, 44, 90, 141
internships 39, 78, 89, 107, 109, 110, 120, 212
interpreters
  business 60–61, 94
  community 53, 54, 85, 142, 215, 233
    see community interpreting 78, 101, 104, 125, 193, 234
  conference 60–61, 83, 94, 97, 98, 105, 203
  dialogue 133, 137
  legal 60–61, 94, 113, 121
  medical xii, xiii, xiv, 1, 2, 3, 4, 5, 6, 11–13, 22, 23, 25, 27, 34, 35, 57, 60, 61, 82, 83, 85, 87, 88, 89, 90, 91, 92, 94, 95, 103, 104, 105, 106, 107, 110, 111, 112, 113, 114, 115, 116, 117, 118, 119, 120, 123, 124, 127, 128, 132, 133, 135, 136, 137, 138, 141, 142, 146, 148, 149, 153, 154, 155, 156, 174, 176, 204, 219
interpreter training xiv, 1, 4, 57, 59, 64, 75, 78, 82, 94, 95, 115, 133, 137, 148, 149, 155, 160
interpreter-facilitators 187, 193, 196, 197
interpreting
  business 69, 70
  conference 70, 75, 77, 78, 80, 82, 86, 87, 88, 92, 94, 95, 97, 101, 115
  consecutive 59, 70, 75, 76, 78–81, 86, 131, 141, 151 *see* consecutive mode 68, 84
  dialogue 69, 70, 71, 72, 75, 84, 86, 90, 96, 99, 101, 104, 108, 141, 153
  healthcare 33, 52, 62, 68, 98, 101, 112, 199, 203 *see* medical xi, xii, xiii, xiv, 2, 3, 4, 5, 6, 9, 10, 11, 21, 22, 24,

Index

27, 33, 38, 52, 57, 58, 59, 60, 61, 62, 64, 68. 69, 70, 71, 72, 75, 77, 82, 83, 87, 88, 89, 90, 94, 95, 96, 97, 103, 104, 105, 106, 107, 108, 109, 111, 112, 115, 119, 120, 121, 122, 123, 124, 127, 128, 129, 131, 135, 136, 137, 139, 141, 144, 153, 154, 156, 157, 165, 166, 175, 181
  in public settings 62, 65, 68 *see* public service (PSI) xii, 59, 62–63, 64, 68, 71, 75, 95, 96, 97, 103, 106
  legal 64, 87, 119
  liaison 62–63, 68, 70, 130
  police 64
  simultaneous 59, 68, 70, 75, 76, 78–81, 86, 131 *see* simultaneous mode 68 *see* simultaneous interpretation 119, 141
  social 63, 70
interpreting services 9, 10, 12, 17, 20, 24, 28, 30, 38, 40, 44, 47, 48, 49, 50, 51, 52, 82, 95, 97, 112, 117, 118, 119, 120, 123
interpreting skills 107, 109, 113, 118, 141, 174
interpreting studies xi, 59, 60, 61
interprofessional xiii, 40, 188, 192
interprofessional education (IPE) xiii
intraprofessional 188, 193

Joint Blended Extracurricular Module on Medical Interpreting 5, 97, 107, 154, 156, 157, 165, 166

language
  access 202, 203, 204, 205, 206, 207, 208, 209, 210, 211, 212, 214, 215, 216
  barriers 31, 35, 119, 124, 202, 205 *see* linguistic barriers 37, 42, 45, 50, 86, 88, 118
  combinations 12, 31, 32, 33, 42, 58, 59, 61, 64, 66, 68, 70, 71, 73, 75, 77, 81, 84, 85, 94, 95, 106, 108, 110, 115, 119, 134, 146, 149
  needs 66, 74, 75, 85
languages of limited diffusion 77, 129
learning
  outcomes 5, 58, 67, 135, 153, 155, 165, 174–175
  platform 2, 4, 5, 84, 97, 128, 129, 131, 132, 133, 138, 139, 153, 155, 159, 161, 166–169, 175, 177
learning-by-doing 193, 194, 195, 197
legislation 3, 6, 10, 11, 15, 16, 17, 20, 21, 22, 23, 24, 28, 49, 52, 74, 93, 109, 111, 112, 113, 115, 119, 167, 206, 212
limited English proficient (LEP) 202 *see also* limited proficiency 17
lingua franca / linguae francae 31, 32, 33, 41, 43, 46, 47, 48, 50, 72, 74, 92, 96, 104, 107, 110, 196
literature review 4, 10, 58

machine translation 44, 97
master's (MA) degree 58, 59, 106 *see* master's level 83
maternity care 158, 171–172
mediation 11, 27, 63, 68, 71, 72, 86, 130
  (inter)cultural 23, 31, 59, 62–65, 68, 69, 70, 71, 72, 76, 79, 86, 87, 96, 108, 119
  linguistic 31, 69, 70, 76, 86, 108 *see also* language mediation 45, 59, 71, 72, 73, 149
  services 25, 26, 31, 32, 37, 38, 40, 51, 119
mediators 11–12, 17, 22, 27, 31, 32, 35, 39, 45, 47, 71, 85, 87, 88, 89, 91, 97 *see* (inter)cultural mediators 22, 23, 24, 26, 27, 31, 45, 59, 71, 74, 85, 86, 108, 109, 112, 115, 118, 119, 124 *see* social/sociocultural mediators 85, 86 see also *mediatori (interculturali)* 22, 69, 108

Medicaid 207, 208
medical terminology 28, 36, 90, 109, 118, 130, 166–167, 174, 176, 177
medical tourism 95, 212
medical translation 59 *see* healthcare translation 63, 66, 68
migrants 1, 23, 32, 58, 72, 73, 74, 75, 84, 86, 89, 96, 108, 177, 188, 211 migrant patients 118, 177 *see also see* migrant population 10, 59, 73, 81 *see* migrant communities 107 *see* migration 71, 75, 81, 130 *see also* immigrants 15, 46, 81, 203, 208, 209, 211, 213 *see also* immigration 44, 59, 60, 75, 86
Ministry
  of Culture 112, 113
  of Education 58 *see* of Education, Culture and Sport (MECD) 58 *see* of Education and Research (MIUR) 59, 69
  of Health 17, 19, 20
  of Justice 113, 119
minority languages 72, 86, 108, 118
monolingual videos 160, 161, 168–173
multi-role roleplays 146, 161, 162, 168–173, 179, 180, 182
multilingual courses 155, 162 *see* multilingual group of students 96 *see* multilingual classes 146

National Health Law Program (NHeLP) 206
new technologies xiv, 18, 118, 211, 213
NGOs 4, 10, 11–13, 14, 23, 25, 26, 32, 33, 86, 93, 105, 118
non-professional interpreters 1, 6, 11–12, 32, 99, 124 *see also* ad hoc interpreters 1, 28, 29, 34, 35, 41, 43, 44, 45, 46, 48, 50, 86, 103, 104, 118, 204

note-taking 63, 68, 131, 146

orthopaedics 134, 135, 136, 144, 158, 170–171, 180, 181

pandemic (COVID-19) 13, 36, 47, 91, 97, 118, 119, 123, 135, 157
Pásalo Project 5, 187, 193, 196
primary care 17, 20, 134
profession 2, 5, 22, 24, 28, 33, 38, 89, 103, 104, 106, 108, 111, 114, 115, 116, 117, 119, 120, 124, 130, 147, 150, 179, 186, 188, 190, 212
professional interpreters 5, 13, 34, 35, 37, 41, 44, 48, 60, 85, 88, 89, 90, 92, 93, 95, 96, 97, 104, 105, 107, 111, 116, 117, 118, 120, 123, 128, 149, 162, 219
professionalization xii, xiii, xiv, 2, 3, 4, 5, 6, 57, 103, 104, 105, 111, 114, 115, 123, 124
psychologically safe space 194, 195
psychotherapy 189, 193

qualifications 22, 23, 24, 59, 106, 207, 211

rates 117, 118, 119, 120, 123, 124
recognition xii, 4, 83, 103, 104, 105, 111, 114, 120, 123
reflective practice 5, 185, 187, 189, 190, 191, 192, 193, 195, 197
refugees 1, 20, 33, 34, 82, 93, 110, 188, 196, 203, 204, 209, 211, 213, 214
remote interpreting xiv, 29, 31, 38, 47, 91, 98, 117, 118, 119, 213
roleplays 72, 90, 91, 134, 135, 143, 144, 145, 146, 161, 162, 163, 168–173, 178, 179, 180, 181, 182

scripted roleplays 96, 140, 143, 144, 161, 162, 163, 168, 170–172, 178,

Index

179, 181 *see also* semi-scripted roleplays 145, 150 *see also* structured roleplays 179v non-scripted/unscripted roleplays 84, 91, 96, 140, 143, 145, 161, 162, 168, 179

Scuole Superiori per Mediatori Linguistici (SSMLs) 69, 70, 108

self-care 153, 158, 172, 173, 175, 176

semi-structured interviews 10, 14 *see* interviews 13, 14, 16, 21, 23, 25, 26, 30, 31, 33, 34, 37, 38, 40, 41, 42, 44, 84

sight translation 68, 69, 84, 90, 131, 134, 137, 141, 142, 146, 160

simulations xiii, xiv, 70, 72, 84, 90, 143, 144

skills xii, xiii, 2, 11–13, 27, 28, 38, 60, 61, 69, 72, 74, 75, 76, 77, 87, 88, 89, 90, 92, 94, 95, 107, 109, 110, 113, 115, 116, 118, 129, 130, 131, 134, 137, 138, 141, 142, 146, 147, 148, 149, 153, 160, 174, 175, 186, 192, 193, 194, 195, 197

social inclusion 2

sociology of professions xii

Socrates method 167, 168, 178

specialization xii, 5, 33, 34, 115, 117, 135

specialized
  care 17
  knowledge xii
  language / terminology /vocabulary 5, 35, 76, 78–79, 83, 135, 147 *see also* medical terminology 28, 36, 90, 109, 118, 130, 166–167, 174, 176, 177
  training xii, 2, 4, 60, 61, 75, 83, 87, 89, 92, 94, 96, 110
  translation 59, 70, 75, 76, 77, 78–81

stakeholders 2, 10, 104

standards 23, 51, 87, 103, 104, 114, 120, 207, 208

stress management 48, 83, 90, 92, 131, 132, 173, 175, 187, 188

support groups 190, 192, 193, 195
syllabi 67, 68, 70

teaching and learning
  materials 3, 5, 159
  practices xiii
tourists 1, 58, 59, 66, 72, 73, 81, 82, 84, 89, 96, 136
training
  methods 61, 91, 95, 121, 128, 141, 142, 143, 149
  resources 4, 5, 97, 114, 127, 128, 129, 131, 133, 136, 153, 182
training modalities 154, 155, 157, 211 *see also* face-to-face training 132, 134, 141, 146, 149, 150, 154, 155, 156, 157, 166 *see also* online training 77, 129, 134, 135, 142, 146, 148, 149, 150, 153, 155, 156, 157, 166, 168 *see also* remote training 97, 141
trauma 83, 109, 113, 123, 132, 173, 187, 188
turn-taking management 84, 174

universities
  Alma Mater Studiorum Università di Bologna (UNIBO) 1, 69, 70, 71, 90
  Universidad de Murcia 1, 63, 66, 107
  Universidad San Jorge (USJ) 1, 63, 66, 94, 107
  Università degli studi Internazionali di Roma (UNINT) 1, 6–70, 71
  Universitatea Babeș-Bolyai (UBB) 1, 76, 79, 109
  Universitatea de Medicină și Farmacie Iuliu Hațieganu 1, 109, 175
university-level programmes 57, 58, 84

working conditions 103, 104, 105, 116, 117, 119, 120, 124, 188
workshops 6, 34, 105, 111, 116, 219

New Trends in Translation Studies

In today's globalised society, translation and interpreting are gaining visibility and relevance as a means to foster communication and dialogue in increasingly multicultural and multilingual environments. Practised since time immemorial, both activities have become more complex and multifaceted in recent decades, intersecting with many other disciplines. *New Trends in Translation Studies* is an international series with the main objectives of promoting the scholarly study of translation and interpreting and of functioning as a forum for the translation and interpreting research community.

This series publishes research on subjects related to multimedia translation and interpreting, in their various social roles. It is primarily intended to engage with contemporary issues surrounding the new multidimensional environments in which translation is flourishing, such as audiovisual media, the internet and emerging new media and technologies. It sets out to reflect new trends in research and in the profession, to encourage flexible methodologies and to promote interdisciplinary research ranging from the theoretical to the practical and from the applied to the pedagogical.

New Trends in Translation Studies publishes translation- and interpreting-oriented books that present high-quality scholarship in an accessible, reader-friendly manner. The series embraces a wide range of publications – monographs, edited volumes, conference proceedings and translations of works in translation studies which do not exist in English. The editor, Professor Jorge Díaz Cintas, welcomes proposals from all those interested in being involved with the series. The working language of the series is English, although in exceptional circumstances works in other languages can be considered for publication. Proposals dealing with specialised translation, translation tools and technology, audiovisual translation and the field of accessibility to the media are particularly welcomed.

Vol. 1   Meng Ji: Phraseology in Corpus-Based Translation Studies
         251 pages. 2010. ISBN 978-3-03911-550-1

Vol. 2   Josu Barambones Zubiria: Mapping the Dubbing
         Scene: Audiovisual Translation in Basque Television
         191 pages. 2012. ISBN 978-3-0343-0281-4

Vol. 3   Elisa Ghia: Subtitling Matters: New Perspectives on Subtitling
         and Foreign Language Learning
         234 pages. 2012. ISBN 978-3-0343-0843-4

Vol. 4   Anabel Borja Albi and Fernando Prieto Ramos (eds): Legal
         Translation in Context: Professional Issues and Prospects
         325 pages. 2013. ISBN 978-3-0343-0284-5

Vol. 5   Kieran O'Driscoll: Retranslation through the Centuries: Jules
         Verne in English
         302 pages. 2011. ISBN 978-3-0343-0236-4

Vol. 6   Federico M. Federici (ed.): Translating Dialects and Languages
         of Minorities: Challenges and Solutions
         245 pages. 2011. ISBN 978-3-0343-0178-7

Vol. 7   Silvia Bruti and Elena Di Giovanni (eds): Audiovisual
         Translation across Europe: An Ever-changing Landscape
         289 pages. 2012. ISBN 978-3-0343-0953-0

Vol. 8   Tong-King Lee: Translating the Multilingual City: Cross-lingual
         Practices and Language Ideology
         176 pages. 2013. ISBN 978-3-0343-0850-2

Vol. 9   Laura Incalcaterra McLoughlin, Marie Biscio and Máire Áine
         Ní Mhainnín (eds): Audiovisual Translation. Subtitles and
         Subtitling: Theory and Practice
         301 pages. 2011. ISBN 978-3-0343-0299-9

Vol. 10   Xiaohui Yuan: Politeness and Audience Response
         in Chinese–English Subtitling
         250 pages. 2012. ISBN 978-3-0343-0732-1

Vol. 11   Isabel García-Izquierdo and Esther Monzó (eds): Iberian
           Studies on Translation and Interpreting
           401 pages. 2012. ISBN 978-3-0343-0815-1

Vol. 12   Claire Ellender: Preserving Polyphonies: Translating the
           Writings of Claude Sarraute
           250 pages. 2013. ISBN 978-3-0343-0940-0

Vol. 13   Pilar Sánchez-Gijón, Olga Torres-Hostench and Bartolomé
           Mesa-Lao (eds): Conducting Research in Translation
           Technologies
           329 pages. 2015. ISBN 978-3-0343-0994-3

Vol. 14   Claire Ellender: Dealing with Difference in Audiovisual
           Translation: Subtitling Linguistic Variation in Films
           221 pages. 2015. ISBN 978-3-0343-1816-7

Vol. 15   Anna Jankowska and Agnieszka Szarkowska (eds): New Points
           of View on Audiovisual Translation and Media Accessibility
           316 pages. 2015. ISBN 978-3-0343-1842-6

Vol. 16   Charlotte Bosseaux: Dubbing, Film and
           Performance: Uncanny Encounters
           251 pages. 2015. ISBN 978-3-0343-0235-7

Vol. 17   Guadalupe Soriano-Barabino: Comparative Law for Legal
           Translators
           220 pages. 2016. ISBN 978-3-0343-1725-2

Vol. 18   Şebnem Susam-Saraeva: Translation and Popular
           Music: Transcultural Intimacy in Turkish–Greek Relations
           184 pages. 2015. ISBN 978-3-03911-887 8

Vol. 19   Celia Martín de León and Víctor González-Ruiz (eds): From
           the Lab to the Classroom and Back Again: Perspectives on
           Translation and Interpreting Training
           371 pages. 2016. ISBN 978-3-0343-1985-0

Vol. 20   Carla Mereu Keating: The Politics of Dubbing: Film Censorship and State Intervention in the Translation of Foreign Cinema in Fascist Italy
191 pages. 2016. ISBN 978-3-0343-1838-9

Vol. 21   Susanne M. Cadera and Andrew Samuel Walsh (eds): Literary Retranslation in Context
252 pages. 2017. ISBN 978-3-0343-1996-6

Vol. 22   Kayoko Nohara: Translating Popular Fiction: Embracing Otherness in Japanese Translations
248 pages. 2018. ISBN 978-3-0343-1963-8

Vol. 23   Pierre-Alexis Mével: Subtitling African American English into French: Can We *Do the Right Thing*?
256 pages. 2017. ISBN 978-3-0343-1897-6

Vol. 24   Micòl Beseghi: Multilingual Films in Translation: A Sociolinguistic and Intercultural Study of Diasporic Films
256 pages. 2017. ISBN 978-1-78707-159-9

Vol. 25   Michal Borodo: Translation, Globalization and Younger Audiences: The Situation in Poland
248 pages. 2017. ISBN 978-1-78707-473-6

Vol. 26   Eugenia Dal Fovo and Paola Gentile (eds): Translation and Interpreting: Convergence, Contact and Interaction
308 pages. 2019. ISBN 978-1-78707-750-8

Vol. 27   Nana Sato-Rossberg and Akiko Uchiyama (eds): Diverse Voices in Translation Studies in East Asia
224 pages. 2019. ISBN 978-178874-022-7

Vol. 28   Sarah M. A. Reed: Translating Cultural Identity: French Translations of Australian Crime Fiction
260 pages. 2019. ISBN 978-1-78874-007-4

Vol. 29   Blanca Arias-Badia: Subtitling Television Series: A Corpus-Driven Study of Police Procedurals
274 pages. 2020. ISBN 978-1-78707-796-6

Vol. 30   Károly Polcz: Speech Acts, Directness and Politeness in
          Dubbing: American Television Series in Hungary
          270 pages. 2020. ISBN 978-1-78874-232-0

Vol. 31   María Dolores Rodríguez Melchor, Ildikó Horváth
          and Kate Ferguson (eds): The Role of Technology in
          Conference Interpreter Training
          262 pages. 2020. ISBN 978-1-78874-407-2

Vol. 32   Ali Almanna and Juan Jose Martinez Sierra (eds):
          Reframing Realities through Translation
          300 pages. 2020. ISBN 978-1-78997-228-3

Vol. 33   Alícia Moreno Giménez: The Translation of Irony: Examining
          its Translatability into Narratives
          262 pages. 2022. ISBN 978-1-78997-984-8

Vol. 34   Esther de Boe: Remote Interpreting in Healthcare Settings
          290 pages. 2023. ISBN 978-1-80079-373-6

Vol. 35   Ali Almanna and Juliane House (eds): Translation Politicised
          and Politics Translated
          268 pages. 2023. ISBN 978-1-80079-446-7

Vol. 36   Carmen Pena-Díaz (ed.): The Making of Accessible
          Audiovisual Translation
          202 pages. 2023. ISBN 978-1-80079-677-5

Vol. 37   Michela Canepari: Specialized Languages and Graphic
          Art: Translating Specialized Discourse Intralingually and
          Intersemiotically
          288 pages. 2023. ISBN 978-1-80079-858-8

Vol. 38   Almudena Nevado Llopis and Ana Isabel Foulquié Rubio (eds):
          Medical Interpreting: Training the Professionals
          266 pages. 2024. ISBN 978-1-80079-321-7

www.ingramcontent.com/pod-product-compliance
Ingram Content Group UK Ltd.
Pitfield, Milton Keynes, MK11 3LW, UK
UKHW021828140426
5217IPUK00017B/1265